# Low-Carb Paleo Diet Recipes

*Top 365 Easy to Cook Low-Carb Paleo Diet Recipes for Breakfast*

JAMES ABRAHAM

# TABLE OF CONTENTS

# Introduction

This book contains proven steps and strategies on how to make paleo breakfasts.

The paleo diet is one of the best functional diets around today. Most people who use it say that the diet has created wonderful changes in their lives. Many people have used this functional diet to lose weight. Athletes also use it to maintain a low body fat percentage and still have the energy to do their activities throughout the day.

This book shows you how you can apply the paleo diet in your breakfast. It gives you 365 ways to prepare paleo meals. The recipes found in this book follow the paleo principle. They are low in calories because these recipes contain very little carbohydrates.

Not only are these recipes excellent to improve your energy level throughout the day, they are also delicious. Start your paleo diet journey today!

We hope the recipes in this book will be able to help you achieve your fitness goals.

# Chapter 1

## All About the Paleo Diet Revolution

Many factors come into play when finding the best functional diet. First, you need to consider your personal goal why you want to modify your diet. Most people do it to lose weight. Other people also use dieting as a way to improve their overall health.

Another factor to consider when dieting is the effects that the nutritional modification has on your body. The best diets make you feel better. Most people however, think that they need to feel starved for a diet to be effective.

When looking for an effective diet, you should also consider the complexity of the principle behind it. A diet should have sound nutritional science background. It should be easy to learn and people's explanation about it should make sense.

Another important factor to consider is the sustainability of the diet. The diet should use ingredients that are available to the individual. The ingredients should also fit the budget of most people.

### What is the paleo diet?

The paleo diet is appealing to most people because it is easy to understand and it makes sense. In this diet, a person aims to eat the way his or her ancestors used to eat when society was still using the hunting and gathering methods to obtain food. In this stage of human civilization, people did not know how to farm. As a result, our ancestors mainly took their energy from foods that they caught and gathered directly from nature.

Foods in this era underwent no processing. Aside from cooking meat, people mostly ate food as they were found in nature. Even the way foods were cooked was different. Our ancestors did not use artificial flavoring. If there was seasoning in some civilizations, they were very minimal and they were mostly done to make the foods last longer. The seasoning ingredients added also undergo very little processing. They should be used as they were found in nature.

Instead of relying on processed food, paleo diet practitioners use whole foods. They also avoid overreliance with carbohydrate staple foods that are produced through industrialized farming.

## Using Paleo diet for breakfast

As most of us have been taught as children, breakfast is one of the most important meals of the day. The food we eat in this part of the day are mostly broken down and used for energy.

Modern humans turn to the most convenient options when preparing breakfast. Because most of us are in a hurry in the morning, we usually neglect to choose the foods with the best nutritional value. Instead, we use easy to prepare processed foods like bacon, chicken nuggets or hotdogs.

With the paleo diet, you will be able to plan your breakfasts so that you maximize the foods' nutritional value. The diet plan should contain recipes that give you the energy that you need while still abiding to the paleo diet rules and guidelines. We will show you these recipes in the next chapter.

# Chapter 2

# Let's start with the Simplest Breakfast Recipes

## Meat and eggs Breakfast

### 1. Hard boiled eggs with spinach

If you want a simple breakfast that you can prepare in less than 30 minutes, just prepare your preferred number of hardboiled eggs, slice them up, and put them on top of a pile of spinach leaves. Use vinaigrette to add flavor to the spinach.

### 2. Scrambled eggs with bacon

Another common and simple recipe is to fry your preferred number of paleo bacon and scramble a pair of eggs. The only difference for paleo practitioners is to use ghee or coconut oil when frying.

### 3. Mushrooms also add great taste to breakfast meats

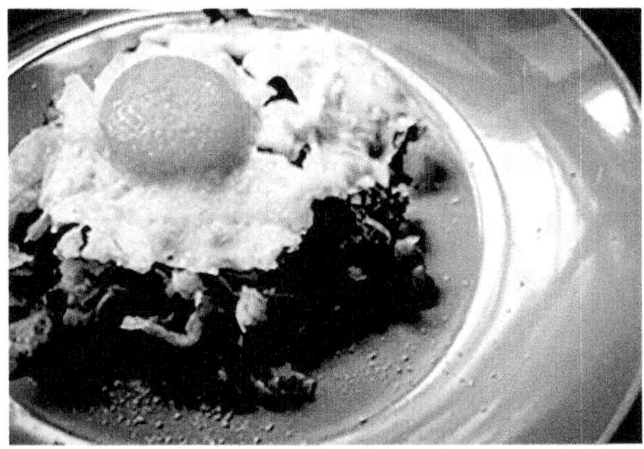

**Photo Source: https://pixabay.com/en/hash-eggs-food-meal-potato-plate-1330575/**

Aside from vegetables, you can also add sautéed mushrooms to your bacon and eggs breakfast.

### 4. Paleo ham with fried eggs and sweet potato

Sweet potato is a low carb alternative to starchy food. You can serve them with ham and fried eggs to add a salty taste. Remember to fry with ghee or coconut oil.

### 5. Paleo ham with scrambled eggs and carrot sticks

If you want to practice paleo diet, you need to become accustomed to eating raw fruits and vegetables. You can start by slicing up some carrot sticks to complement with your ham and eggs.

### 6. Bacon, eggs and fresh fruits

Most types of meat and eggs recipe are dry if you do not add vegetables and fruits into the mix. You can add fruits like papaya to the bacon and egg duo to add some moisture to your food.

### 7. Bacon, eggs and berries

You may also add berries to the mix. Fresh berries are always better than preserved ones. The same goes with fruits. Berries also add some moisture to your meals.

### 8. Use coconut and almond milk instead of dairy

If you want some milky flavor in your breakfast, the paleo diet does not use dairy milk. Instead, you should use coconut milk and almond milk. In some tropical countries, these are sold fresh. For most people however, we may need to use canned versions.

### 9. Bacon, hard boiled eggs and spinach salad

You will also be able to prepare an easy meal of bacon, hard-boiled eggs and spinach in the morning. You can use vinaigrette to give flavor to the spinach. You will also need it because the bacon is not processed with salt or sweeteners.

### 10. Add salads to your bacon and egg breakfasts

You can enhance the vitamin content of all your meat and egg breakfasts by serving them with the salads suggested in this book.

### 11. Meat, Eggs and steamed vegetables

You can also add vegetables to your meat and eggs by adding steamed vegetables to it. Steam some broccoli, carrots and peas and add them to your breakfast.

### 12. Sautéed vegetable with meat and eggs

Aside from fresh and steamed vegetables, you can also sauté them to add flavor. Ideally, you should use a variety of ways to cook your vegetables.

# Chapter 3

# Paleo Breakfast Salads

**Paleo salads:**

1. **Paleo Kale Breakfast Salad**

## Ingredients:

- 2 cups avocado
- 3 tsps. freshly squeezed lemon juice
- 4 tsps. olive oil
- 1 tsp. cayenne pepper
- 1 cup red onion
- 4 strips of bacon
- 500 grams of kale head
- Sea salt (to taste)

## Instructions:

a. Dice the avocadoes, onions and tomatoes. Remove the ribs from the kale and chop the leaves. Put them in a mixing bowl.

b. In a pan, fry the bacon in its own fat for 4-5 minutes. It should be crispy enough to be chopped or broken into smaller pieces. Add them to the mixing bowl.

c. Add all other listed ingredients to the bowl. Toss them all with a ladle. Massage the kale and the avocado to soften the leaves.

d. Let the tossed salad sit for 15 minutes to allow the flavors to blend.

Serves 8-12

**2. The chard variation**

Chard also tastes good with this recipe. You can use it to replace kale if it is not available in your area.

**3. The collard greens variation**

Collard also works well if it is more abundant in your area. ½ cup of this green vegetable will add 25 calories to your salad with 3 grams of fibers. It also contains Vitamins A and C.

**4. The lettuce variation**

You can create the above ingredients with lettuce instead of kale. You should avoid pressing it though to maintain the crunchiness.

**5. The apples and pears variety**

If you want some crunchy fruits with your salad, you can add slices of apples and pears without the core to the mix.

**6. The spinach variation**

You can also choose to use spinach. Instead of adding its leaves to the salad, you should mix all the other ingredients first and add them on top of the spinach leaves.

**7. The Bacon and Greens version**

Regardless of the types of greens you use, you can add salty and meaty flavors to your salad by adding more fired bacon. In our recipe, we used 4 strips of bacon. You can double it to 8 if you want to increase the caloric content of your dish.

**8. Turkey Bacon with greens version**

You can also use turkey bacon instead of pork bacon. Use this if you want to minimize the amount of fat in your dish.

**9. Macon with greens version**

If you live in an area with a lot of sheep, there is a good chance that you have access to Macon. Macon is bacon made from mutton.

**10. Vegetarian bacon and greens variation**

If you want this dish to be 100% vegetarian you may use vegetarian bacon as an alternative to bacon.

**11. Kale salad with hard boiled eggs**

You can also add cut up hardboiled eggs to your salad if you want to add more protein into it.

**12. Serve with grilled chicken breasts if you need protein**

Most paleo diet practitioners follow the diet for improved work or sports performance. If you want the same results, you should add simple grilled chicken breasts seasoned with salt and ground pepper to this salad recipe.

**13. Paleo Spinach Breakfast Salad**

## Ingredients:

- 4 eggs
- 2 red onions
- 2 cups fresh basil
- 4 cups baby spinach
- 4 tbsp. black olives
- 6 tbsp. olive oil

- 2 tbsp. fresh oregano
- 2/3 cup freshly squeezed lemon juice
- 2 avocadoes

**Instructions:**

a) Prepare the ingredients by chopping the red onion, basil, oregano and black olives. Peel, pit and dice the avocado.

b) Boil the egg until hard. When it is cool enough, peel and chop it.

c) Add all the ingredients in a large bowl and toss.

Serves 6-8 people

### 14. Use baby arugula as an alternative

If there is low supply of baby spinach, there may be a need to replace it with baby arugula. This green leafy vegetable is the closest to baby spinach but it also has a mustard-like tinge.

### 15. Baby lettuce version

You may also try this recipe using baby lettuce instead of spinach. The texture and the taste of the greens will be completely different. However, you can still do it to add a variety to your meals.

### 16. Watercress variation

You can also make use of watercress as the primary greens to add variety.

### 17. Paleo Spinach Breakfast Salad with Hard boiled eggs

Most people may want to add more protein to their salads. In this case, you may add sliced hard-boiled eggs to the mix to add more mass to your meal.

### 18. Paleo Spinach Breakfast Salad with apples

You can add a crunchy texture to the salad by adding apples to the salad. Slice them, remove the core and the seeds and add them to the mix.

### 19. Salad using 4 types of leaves

You may also choose to use 2-4 types of leaves when making this salad. You can use a portion of baby spinach, baby arugula, baby lettuce and watercress.

### 20. Serve with grilled chicken breast

You may also consider adding grilled chicken breast. You can grill chicken breasts with other vegetables like tomatoes and Brussels sprouts. Serve them with this salad recipe.

### 21. Using vinaigrette instead of olive oils

You can also choose to use your preferred brand of vinaigrette instead of the olive oil. You should make sure however, that you choose the ones with minimal sugar content.

### 22. Curried Breakfast Salad

## Ingredients:

- 1 kg. chicken breast (skinless, boneless)
- 1 cup Paleo mayonnaise
- ½ cup dried apricots
- ¼ cup dried cranberries
- 1 Gala apple (small)
- 4 tbsp. chives
- 1 celery stalk
- 2 tbsp. scallion

- 2 small red onions
- 2 tsp. curry powder
- Salt and pepper to taste
- 2 avocadoes

**Instructions:**

a. Cook the chicken and dice the meat.

b. Prepare the ingredients by mincing the apricots, cranberries, chives, white part of the scallion and red onions. Dice the avocadoes, apple and the celery stalk.

c. Put all the prepared ingredients in a mixing bowl and add pepper or salt to taste.

Serves 6-8 people

## 23. Vegan Variation

Instead of using chicken, you can also substitute it with tofu. You should also cook the tofu to make it firmer. Dice it and add it to the dish as you would with the chicken.

## 24. Curried Breakfast Salad with spinach

If you are on a mission to add green leafy vegetables to your breakfast, you can also add spinach to this dish.

## 25. Curried Breakfast Salad with lettuce

You can also add a lettuce in a bowl with vinaigrette and tomatoes. The tomatoes should be halved or quartered depending on the size.

## 26. Replace the apples with pears

Gala apples may not be abundant in some places. If this is the case, it can be replaced with more common types of fruits like pears. Pears taste great raw with most types of salads.

### 27. Double avocado version

Most people who love avocados should add more than the prescribed amount. If you enjoy avocadoes in your salad, you may also double the amount. This will add a more pasty and milky taste to the salad.

### 28. Curry salad with eggs

You may also make this salad more protein-rich by adding poached eggs on top of it.

### 29. Replace Chicken with tofu

If you are on a meat free paleo diet, you can also replace the chicken with tofu. You may fry the tofu with ghee or melted coconut oil.

### 30. Curry salad with spicy tofu

You can also make the curried tofu salad more interesting by adding sliced and deseeded jalapenos. If this is too spicy, just add a pinch of paprika.

### 31. Chicken Breakfast Salad with mangoes

**Ingredients:**

- 4 pieces large chicken breasts (boneless, skinless)
- 4 scallions
- 1 ½ large fennel bulb
- ½ cup Fresh parsley
- 4 cups baby spinach
- 3 large mangoes (Approximately ½ kilo)
- 2 avocadoes
- Sweet vinaigrette to taste

**Instructions:**

a. Prepare the ingredients by grilling and chopping the chicken. Chop the fennel until fine. You should also chop the scallion to bitesize pieces.

b. Peel the mangoes and the avocadoes and remove the seeds. Scrape their pulp. Dice the avocadoes and chop the mango pulp.

c. Add the fennel, chicken, scallion and parsley in a mixing bowl and mix.

d. Divide the mixture into 6 plates. Divide the spinach into the same number of servings and put it on top of the chicken-fennel mixture. Add the chopped avocadoes and mangoes on top.

Serves 6 people

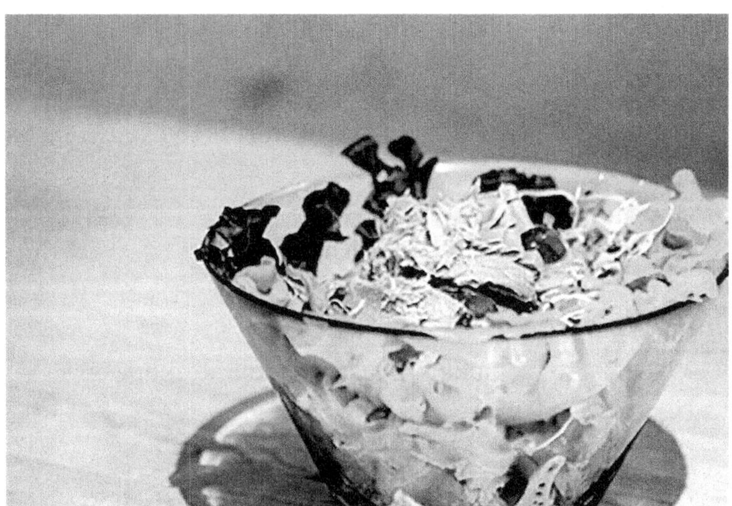

**Photo Source: https://pixabay.com/en/salad-tuna-salad-article-nafut-1088411/**

### 32. Using tofu instead of chicken

Just like with the previous chicken recipe, you can also replace the chicken with tofu.

### 33. Banana alternative for mangoes

Mangoes are the best option for this salad. However, in certain parts of the year, they may be in low supply. As an alternative, you can use sliced bananas.

### 34. Papaya substitute for mangoes

Ripe papayas have a different smell and their pulp is dry. Other than that, their texture closely resembles to that of mangoes. This makes them a good substitute for mangoes when the latter is not in season.

### 35. Nectarine alternative for mangoes

Nectarine also tastes great and its texture and smell are similar to mangoes. You can use this fruit in this recipe as well to replace mangoes.

### 36. Using peaches instead of mangoes

Peaches also work well as a mango alternative. They have a stronger smell but they are more available in some places.

### 37. Use multiple fruits instead of just one

If you want a sweet tasting paleo meal in the morning, you can just use multiple types of fruits in this dish. The chicken or tofu will neutralizes the sweetness so you should also increase the amount of meat.

### 38. Serve with fried eggs

If your chicken and fruit salad may seem lacking in protein, you may add eggs fried with ghee to the mix.

### 39. Replace vinaigrette with olive oil

If the sweet vinaigrette is too sweet for the fruits, you may choose to replace it with virgin olive oil. Squeeze half a lemon into the salad to add a tangy taste to the olive oil.

### 40. Breakfast Crab Salad

**Ingredients**:

- Pepper and sea salt to taste
- 3 tbsp. Paleo mayonnaise
- 2 tbsp. freshly squeezed lemon juice
- 1 kg. lump crab meat (Drained and cleaned for broken shell)
- 3 scallions
- 3 tbsp. fresh parsley (Italian)

**Instructions:**

a. Slice the scallions thinly. Mince the Italian parsley. Steam the crabmeat.

b. Add all ingredients in a bowl. Mix thoroughly. Add the salt and pepper to taste.

Serves 6 people

### 41. Using avocadoes instead of mayonnaise

If you want an organic substitute to commercially sold paleo mayonnaise, you can use avocados. You should mash the avocadoes into the right consistency. You should then add sea salt and ground pepper to taste.

### 42. Surimi substitute for crab meat

You can also use starch-less surimi as an alternative for crabmeat. It is still paleo because they are made of common fish meat like cod.

### 43. Monkfish alternative

Monkfish also perfectly mimics the texture of crabmeat. You can use it if it is common in your area.

### 44. Tuna alternative for crab

If crab is too expensive in your area and the other suggestions are not easily available, you can also use canned tuna in water. The taste will be different but it will give you the necessary seafood flavor.

### 45. Egg-enriched crab meat

If you want a tastier crabmeat, you should scramble it with eggs before mixing it with the rest of the ingredients. This will cover the meat with coating of eggs. Use ghee when frying.

### 46. Add spinach for fiber

You can add more bulk to this meal without adding calories by adding leafy-greens like spinach.

### 47. Kale and crab salad

You can also use kale. You should use more of the dressing if you want to use more leafy greens.

### 48. Serve the leafy greens in a different bowl

You can also choose to serve the leafy-greens in a separate bowl with vinaigrette and olive oil. Just eat them together.

### 49. Wrap the salad in lettuce

If you cut up allingredients thinly, you can eat the crab salad using lettuce wraps. Serve the salad with individual lettuce leaves. When eating it, you should spoon the salad into the lettuce surface and wrap the leaf around it.

### 50. Tuna Salad for Breakfast

**Ingredients:**

- ½ cups wild caught tuna (steamed)
- 7 tbsp. Olive Oil Mayo
- Mustard powder to taste
- Salt and pepper to taste
- 1 large Fuji apple
- 3 scallions
- 3 tbsp. pecans

**Instructions:**

a. Prepare the ingredients by dicing the apple and slicing the scallions into thin strips. Chop the tuna. Chop the pecans and mince the parsley.

b. Mix the apple, nuts, scallions and parsley in a bowl and mix them with a fork.

c. Add the tuna.

d. Add ½ teaspoon of mustard powder and mayo to the bowl and blend them with a spatula.

e. Let the mixture sit for 10 minutes. Adjust the taste with mustard powder, salt and pepper.

Serves 3 people

### 51. The canned tuna version

You can also do the above recipe using canned tuna. You should make sure however, that you use tuna chunks in water. When adding the tuna to the salad, you should break the chunks up into smaller pieces.

### 52. Serve with scrambled eggs on the side

We have a few of side dishes in our selection of dishes in this book. You may choose from any of them to complement your tuna breakfast. The simplest way however, is to serve it with scrambled eggs.

### 53. Using peaches as an apple alternative

Peaches also work great as an apple alternative for this dish. It also tastes great with the mustard powder, olive oil, mayo, and salt.

### 54. Using almonds instead of pecan

You can also choose to use slivered almonds instead of pecan. In some places, almonds are a cheaper source. You should consider however, that pecans have a stronger taste than almonds.

### 55. Serve with spinach

When serving this salad, first put your desired amount of spinach on the plate. Then, put the mound of tuna salad on top of it.

### 56. Add assorted nuts for a nutty flavor

You can also add unsalted assorted nuts to add a crunchy texture to the salad. Crush them with a rolling pin before adding them to the salad mix.

### 57. Eat with lettuce wraps

Just like the crabmeat salad, you can also eat this salad with lettuce wraps. You should slice the apples and other large ingredients thinly to make sure they will fit the lettuce.

# Chapter 4

# More Egg Recipes

### 58. Sweet potatoes and eggs breakfast

## Ingredients:

- 3 cups diced sweet potatoes
- 10 medium eggs
- ½ cup almond milk
- 2 green onions
- 3 tsp. chili powder
- 3 tsp. dried oregano
- 1 cup fresh salsa
- 3 tbsp. ghee
- Sea salt and pepper to taste

## Instructions:

a. Dice the sweet potatoes and slice the green onions into thin slices.

b. Prepare a pot of water and heat it until it is almost boiling. Cook sweet potatoes in it for 8 minutes.

c. In a bowl, add the eggs, oregano, almond milk and chili powder. Mix the ingredients and add the seasoning ingredients to taste.

d. In a medium-high heat, melt the ghee in a skillet and add the egg mixture. Stir and cook until the eggs have settled

e. Divide the potatoes into six servings and place them in a plate. Add the egg mixture on top of it and top it with salsa and green onion slices.

### 59. Using coconut milk instead of almond milk

If you want to lessen the nutty flavor from this dish, you may choose to use coconut milk instead of almond milk.

### 60. Pearled barley alternative for potatoes

Pearled barley is also a low carb alternative to sweet potato. Some people just do not like the taste of this root crop. If you feel the same way, you should also try using pearl barley for this recipe.

### 61. Serve with turkey breakfast sausage

This is one of the recipes in this book with some starch in it. This will taste great if served with the turkey breakfast sausage discussed later in the book.

### 62. Increase the chili powder to make it more spicy

If you want your breakfast to be spicier, increase the amount of chili powder. Add 5 teaspoons instead of the 3 suggested above.

### 63. Serve with raw spinach

You can also add raw spinach to add a crunchy texture to the meal. You may serve the spinach in a separate bowl with vinaigrette.

### 64. Add bacon bits

If you want more protein and fat content, you may also add fried and cut-up bacon to the mix. This will add a salty taste to the dish.

### 65. Use turkey bacon instead of pork bacon

If you are conscious of the fat content of the meal, you can replace pork bacon bits with turkey bacon. It will still add a meaty flavor to your sweet potato dish.

### 66. Paleo Cinnamon Pancake Breakfast

## Ingredients:

- 2 large eggs
- 5 tbsp. coconut milk
- 5 tbsp. ripe banana
- 1 tsp. apple cider vinegar
- 1 tsp. vanilla extract
- 2 ½ tbsp. coconut flour
- 1 tsp. ground cinnamon
- ½ tsp. baking soda
- ¼ tsp. sea salt
- 2 tbsp. ghee

## Instructions:

a. Add the eggs, coconut milk, vinegar, banana and vanilla in a bowl. Mash the banana with all the other ingredients and mix them all together.

b. In another bowl, add the salt, baking soda, cinnamon and flour. Mix them together.

c. Combine the contents of the two bowls. The mixture should have a thin consistency. If the batter is two thick, add a proportionate amount of the wet ingredients.

d. Heat the ghee in a frying pan at medium heat. Add the batter to make pancake shapes.

e. Cook the first side until the edges start to become golden. Flip and cook the other side for about 45 seconds.

Serves 3-4 people

### 67. The Banana-Mango Version

If you want to add more flavor to your pancakes, you may also add a spoonful of mashed mango pulp in the batter. Leave some pulp as a syrup alternative.

### 68. Bacon and apple pancakes

If you remove the cinnamon from the ingredients, you get a basic paleo pancake recipe. You can add virtually anything to this basic recipe. For instance, you can add cut-up bacon with grated apple to the batter to make bacon and apple pancakes.

### 69. Use cacao nibs to the batter

If you want a strong chocolatey flavor to your cinnamon pancake, you can add cacao nibs to the batter.

### 70. Pear and apple variation

You can also change the apple to an equal number of pears because they may be more abundant in certain parts of the year.

### 71. Add shredded coconut meat to add texture

If fresh coconuts are available in your area, you can add shredded coconut meat to the batter. This will add more texture to the pancakes.

### 72. Add ham and eggs for a complete breakfast

You can serve this dish with ham and scrambled eggs or frittatas to make your breakfast complete.

### 73. Use raw honey for syrup

If you are thinking of Paleo syrup for your pancakes, raw honey is the best option.

### 74. Serve with breakfast sausages

You will find many breakfast sausage recipes later in the book. Choose one from among them to serve with your fruity pancake. The turkey breakfast sausage is the best one to start with.

### 75. Paleo Banana Pancakes with almonds

- 3 eggs
- 6 ripe bananas
- 2 tbsp. almond butter
- 2tbsp. ghee

## Instructions:

a. Mash the bananas in a bowl. Add the eggs and mix them together.

b. Add the almond butter and stir.

c. Melt the ghee in low heat and then pour the batter to make the pancake.

d. Cook each side until brown.

Serves 4 people

### 76. Paleo banana pancakes with nectarine

If you want your banana pancakes to be sweeter, you may also choose to add mashed nectarine pulp into the mix before cooking. You can also use candied nectarine as the syrup.

### 77. Serve with apples

Instead of eating your banana pancakes without a side, slice up a few apples of your choice to go along with it. This will add a whole food that will increase your chewing frequency, which is important in the paleo diet.

### 78. Cherry topped banana pancakes

Your banana pancakes will taste great with the addition of cherries on top of it. Make some cherry-sugar syrup. All you have to do is to boil the cherries with ¼-cup sugar and 1 tablespoon of water. You should then use this syrup for your banana pancakes.

### 79. Flaxseed and strawberry pancake variation

You can also add variety to your diet by adding mashed blueberries to your pancakes instead of the mashed bananas. You can even add a sprinkle of flax seeds when mixing the batter.

### 80. Banana pancakes with pear on the side

You can also serve banana pancakes with slices of pear to add a whole food to your meal. This is a good substitute to apples for variety.

### 81. Cocoa Banana pancakes

When mixing the batter, you should add 1 tablespoon of cocoa butter to add a chocolate flavor to the pancakes.

### 82. Strawberries and lemon juice pancake

You can also add a citrusy smell to the pancake by adding 1 teaspoon of lemon juice to it. Enhance the experience by adding slices of strawberries when serving it.

## 83. Paleo Raspberry Pancakes

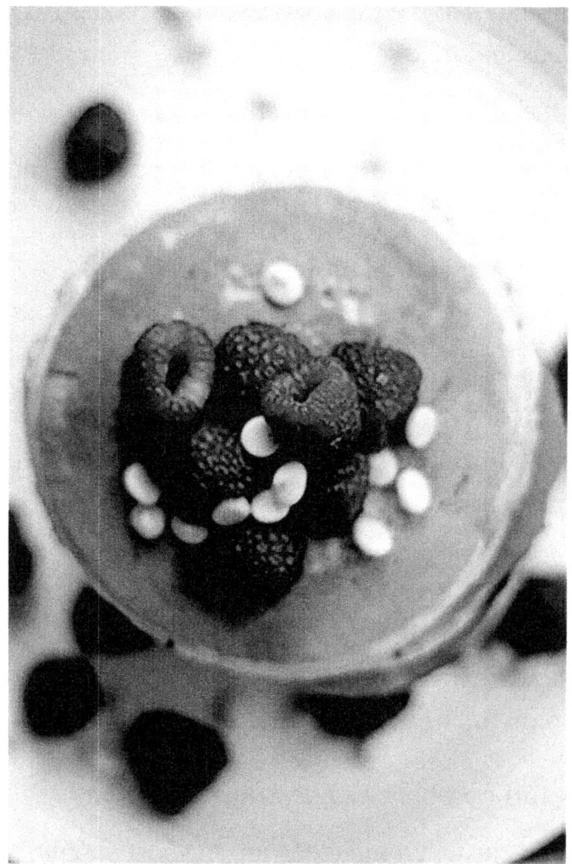

**Photo Source: https://pixabay.com/en/pancakes-raspberries-fruits-925482/**

## Ingredients:

- 3 eggs
- ½ cup Banana
- 1 cup of raspberries
- 2 tbsp. almond butter
- 2tbsp. grass-fed butter

**Instructions:**

a. Mash half of the raspberries in a bowl. Add the eggs, bananas and mix.

b. Add the almond butter and stir.

c. Melt the butter in low-heat and then pour the batter to make the pancake circles

d. Cook each side until brown.

Serves 4 people

### 84. Mangoes and raspberries pancakes variation

You can also add mashed mango pulp to the batter of the pancakes. The fresh raspberries should neutralize the sweetness of the mangoes.

### 85. Avocado and raspberry pancakes

You can also add avocados to this version of pancakes. Mash them and add them on top of the pancakes when serving with syrup.

### 86. Peach and raspberries pancakes variations

In parts of the year when mangoes are in short supply, you can use peaches to replace them.

### 87. Assorted berries pancakes

You can also use assorted berries as a substitute for this recipe and any of its variations. Most berries become abundant during middle and late spring. You will have many berries to choose from at this time of the year.

### 88. Serve with coconut cream

Raspberry pancakes taste great with coconut cream. Make sure you use paleo brands.

### 89. Top with bacon bits

To add protein to your pancakes, break apart 3-4 pieces of crisp-fried bacon and add them on top of the coconut cream.

### 90. Paleo Omelet

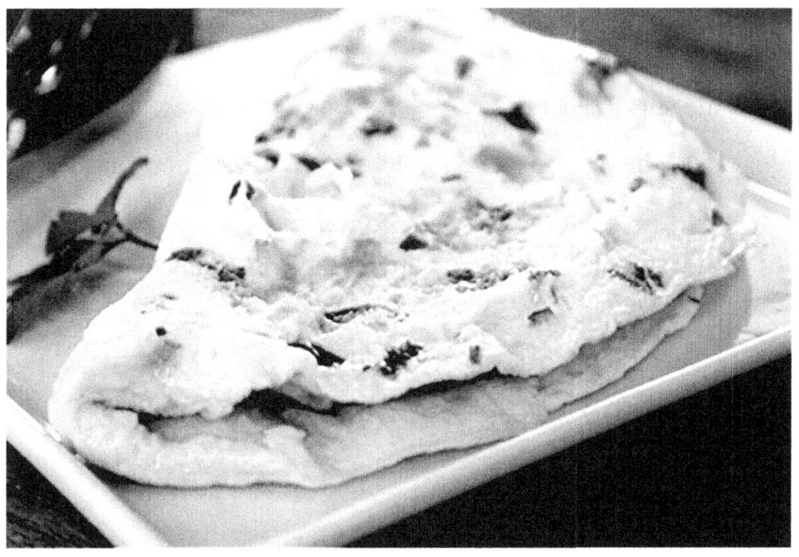

**Photo Source: https://pixabay.com/en/kitchen-omelet-eggs-food-healthy-775746/**

## Ingredients:

- 8 eggs
- 2 tsp. fish sauce
- 4 tbsp. fresh cilantro
- 4 tbsp. scallions
- 1 whole Lime
- 1 tbsp. ghee

## Instructions:

a. Chop the cilantro and scallions. Slice the lime into four.

b. Add the eggs into a bowl. Add the sauce, chopped cilantro and scallions. Squeeze the lime wedges to extract the juices.
c. Whisk the ingredients together until froth bubbles begin to show.
d. Heat the ghee in high heat using a cast iron skillet. Cover the whole skillet with the melted ghee by swirling it around the surface.
e. Add the egg mixture and let it cook for 10 seconds.
f. Tilt the skillet to one side to make the uncooked egg bunch to one side. Using a spatula, flip the thinner size over the other side.
g. Remove the omelet from the heat if satisfied with the consistency.

Serves 2 people

### 91. Paleo Omelet with Broccoli center

You can also make your omelet even more special by adding bits of broccoli inside it. To do this, you should cut your broccoli into thin pieces. You should then put them on top of your omelet before folding it.

### 92. Paleo Omelet with Bacon and Tomatoes

You can also use bacon and tomatoes as your omelet filling. You should fry the bacon as instructed earlier in the book. The tomatoes on the other hand, should be chopped. Add the fried bacon and chopped tomatoes before folding the omelet.

### 93. Chili and non-dairy cheese omelet

You can also do a chili and cheese variation of the omelet recipe above if you want your breakfast to make you sweat. You should make sure however, that you use non-dairy cheese.

### 94. Smoked salmon Omelet

You can also add more protein to your omelet by adding sliced smoked salmon into the mix. Add dill and capers for more flavors.

### 95. Fresh basil omelet

You can also add fresh basil to the omelet. This will add a strong aroma to your omelet.

### 96. Spinach Omelet

You can also add spinach as your filling to the omelet. However, you should also add chopped onions, tomatoes and mushrooms.

### 97. Spinach, bacon and mashed cashew

Aside from onions and tomatoes, you can also use bacon and mashed cashew to make your spinach omelet tastier. It also adds more protein to your diet.

### 98. Onion and mushroom

On days when you are on a hurry, you can also add this simple pair to your omelet, chopped onion and mushroom. You should sauté the pair before adding them to your omelet.

### 99. Wild salmon omelet

Enhance the protein content of your omelet by adding fish meat into it. To make this happen, you should sauté two ounces of salmon with one diced green onion. You should then add this sauté mix to the omelet as a filling.

### 100. Bacon avocado omelet

Bacon and avocadoes are also excellent fillings for your omelet. You should cook the bacon first until crispy. You should then cut it up into multiple pieces. You should also dice the avocadoes. Add them to the omelet just before you fold it.

### 101. Mushroom with watercress omelet

If you want something soft and crunchy inside your omelet, add mushrooms and watercress. You should first, sauté the mushroom in olive oil and garlic. Add the watercress directly together with the sautéed mushrooms.

### 102. Post-Thanksgiving omelet

If you have leftover turkey during thanksgiving, you should also consider dicing its meaty parts and adding it to your omelet as a filling. Mix them with fried bacon to add flavor.

### 103. Mushrooms and asparagus omelet

Sautéed mushrooms taste great with omelet. Sauté fresh mushrooms using coconut oil and garlic. You should also add 3-4 steamed asparagus spears.

### 104. Paleo Scrambled Eggs with Broccoli

**Ingredients:**

- 2 ½ tbsp. ghee
- Pinch of salt and pepper
- 3 cups broccoli (Chopped)
- ½ cup red onion (Chopped)
- 9 eggs
- 1 tsp. dried oregano
- Pinch of Cayenne pepper

**Instructions:**

a. Heat the skillet at low for 1 and ½ minutes and add the ghee. Add the pinch of salt and pepper.

b. When the ghee has totally melted, add broccoli and onions. Increase the heat to medium-high. Sauté the broccoli and onions for 1-1 ½ minutes.

c. In a medium bowl, add the oregano, cayenne and eggs and mix them well. Decrease the heat to medium before adding the egg and spice mixture into the skillet.

d. Let the egg and broccoli cook undisturbed for a few seconds.

e. With a spatula, slightly flip or stir the mixture. Take the dish out of the fire before the eggs totally dry out.

f. Divide the scrambled egg to the number of dishes.

Serves 6-8 people

## 105. Paleo Scrambled Eggs with Broccoli and Avocadoes

You can even improve the recipe above by garnishing with avocadoes. Slice one large avocado, remove its seed, scrape the pulp and dice it. Add the diced avocados on top of your broccoli dish.

## 106. Paleo Scrambled Eggs with Broccoli and Strawberries

During strawberry season, you can also make the strawberry variation of the dish. You should slice the strawberries into three or four bitesize pieces. Add them as a flavorful garnish on top of the broccoli dish.

### 107. Paleo Scrambled Eggs with Spinach

Aside from using broccoli, you should also consider adding spinach to your scrambled eggs. You should scramble the eggs without the broccoli and then add the eggs on top of piles of spinach leaves on the plate.

### 108. Cauliflower as a broccoli alternative

Cauliflower may not taste the same but they offer similar texture to broccoli. Use it as a substitute if broccolis are not available.

### 109. Paleo Scrambled Eggs with diced tomatoes

Adding diced tomatoes to the mix will give a soft moist texture to the scrambled eggs.

### 110. Paleo Scrambled Eggs with breakfast sausage bits

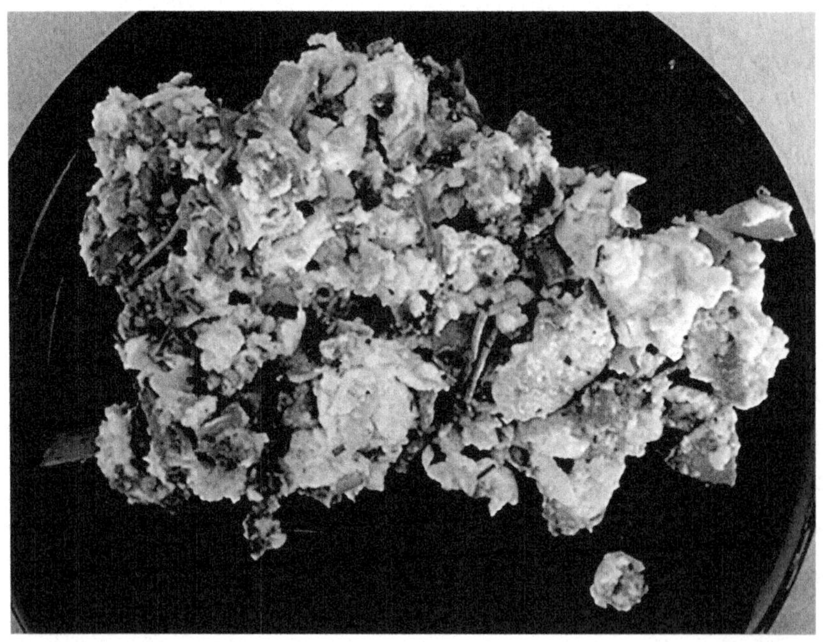

**Photo Source: https://pixabay.com/en/scrambled-eggs-breakfast-fried-eat-6128/**

Refer to the sausage recipes in the later part of this book. Cut up the cooked sausages and sprinkle them on top of the scrambled egg.

### 111. Replace broccoli with kale

You can replace the broccoli with kale. However, you should add them fresh after cooking the scrambled eggs. They are better eaten fresh.

### 112. Scrambled eggs with sausage and vegetables

## Ingredients:

- 10 eggs
- Cooked and sliced Paleo turkey sausage
- 1 cup chopped broccoli
- 7 tbsp. full-fat coconut milk
- Pinch of salt and pepper
- Ghee for frying

## Instructions:

a. Mix the coconut milk, eggs, salt, and pepper in a bowl and whisk.

b. Heat the skillet in low heat and add the ghee. Add the broccoliwhen the ghee has covered the pan surface and stir. Add the egg mixture.

c. Add the sausage slices on top of the eggs. When some of the eggs are cooked, start to scramble the eggs with a spatula by stirring the solid ones with the liquid parts of the egg.

Serves 4-6 people

### 113. Leftover ham variation

You do not have to use paleo turkey sausage for this recipe. Any prepared meat that counts as paleo can be added to the mixture. Make sure to precook meat types that are still raw. For instance, use some of your prosciutto ham leftover from other recipes.

### 114. Spinach variation

You can also change the types of leafy vegetables that you use. For example, use spinach instead of broccoli. Cook the eggs without the spinach and pour the scrambled egg over fresh spinach when serving.

### 115. Bacon variation

You can also use bacon to add flavor to your scrambled eggs. You should precook the bacon to a crispy consistency. Cut them up to smaller pieces and add them as you would add the sausage slices.

### 116. Ground beef variation

You may choose to add ground beef instead to add more protein to your breakfast meal. Cook the ground beef on another pan and add it to the eggs when you are about to serve.

### 117. Ground pork variation

The ground pork variation of this recipe will taste great but it adds more fat. Use the same instructions with the ground beef variation.

### 118. Scrambled eggs with spicy sausage

You can also choose to add spicy sausage to your scrambled eggs recipe.

# Chapter 5

# Unique Paleo Fruit and Vegetable Dishes

### 119. Paleo Italian Broccoli Breakfast Sides

## Ingredients:

- ½ cup coconut oil
- 3 cloves crushed garlic
- 4 medium sized tomatoes (Diced and boiled into a broth)
- 1 ½ tbsp. balsamic vinegar
- ½ tbsp. dried basil leaves
- 2 lbs. broccoli, cut into long spears
- Salt and pepper to taste

## Instructions:

a. In a skillet, heat the coconut oil over medium heat.

b. Cook the garlic first for a few minutes and let the flavor come out by stirring it regularly.

c. Add the tomato, vinegar, and basil. Let the tomato soup simmer until a third of the liquid has evaporated.

d. Add the broccoli on top of the tomato. Add salt and pepper to taste.

e. Make the broccoli become tender by cooking it at low heat for 8-10 minutes.

Serves 6 people

120. **Paleo Italian Green Cabbage Breakfast Sides**

121. **Green cabbage can be a good substitute. When making this substitute however, be careful not to overcook the cabbage by adjusting the cooking time.**

## 122. Nutty Cauliflower Breakfast Sides

Using the instructions above, you can also replace the broccoli with cauliflower. Because the taste of cauliflower is not as strong as broccoli's, you should also change the coconut oil for macadamia nut oil. This will enhance the flavor of the breakfast side dish.

123. **Paleo Sautéed Kohlrabi breakfast sides**

### Ingredients:

- 4 Kohlrabies
- 2 tbsp. ghee
- 4 cloves crushed garlic
- Salt and pepper to taste

### Instructions:

a. Remove the stalks and the bottom from the kohlrabies. After peeling the bulb, cut them into thin slices.

b. Boil water in a pot, add the vegetables, and cook until it is firm. If the firmness is just right, drain them and run them through running water.

c. Heat the ghee in a pan and add the crushed garlic. Sauté the garlic until it is golden brown. Add the boiled kohlrabies and a pinch of salt and pepper. Sauté until golden brown.

Serves 6 people

### 124. Broccoli stems variation

You may substitute kohlrabies with broccoli stems if the vegetable is not common in your country.

### 125. White radish version

Though the taste will become stronger, you can change the kohlrabies with white radish. You can make this substitute if you want your breakfast sides to have a stronger taste.

### 126. Turnip substitute

You can substitute the kohlrabies with turnips. It is a more common vegetable so use it in seasons with low kohlrabi supply.

### 127. Paleo honey muffins

## Ingredients:

- 4 eggs
- 4 tbsp. honey
- 3 tbsp. macadamia nut oil
- 3 tbsp. fresh coconut milk
- ½ tsp. salt
- ½ tsp. vanilla extract
- ½ tsp. baking powder
- ½ cup coconut flour
- 2 mashed ripe banana

## Instructions:

a. Preheat the oven to 200 degrees Celsius. In 6 muffin cups, place the paper liners.

b. Add the egg, oil, honey, salt, coconut milk and vanilla to a bowl and mix.

c. In a separate bowl, mix the baking powder with the coconut flour before adding it to the wet mixing bowl.
d. Add the mashed banana and mix thoroughly. Divide it to the prepared muffin cups and cook.

Serves 8 people

### 128. Honey muffins with chopped pecans

You can enhance the texture and the flavors even more by mixing in chopped pecans when mixing.

### 129. Paleo Honey Strawberry muffins

You can also replace the mashed bananas with chopped fresh strawberries for a different flavored muffin.

### 130. Walnuts honey strawberry muffins

On top of replacing bananas with strawberries, you can also add walnuts when mixing. This will add the nutty texture to your muffins and enhance its taste.

### 131. Hickory nuts honey muffin

Regardless of what fruit you choose, you can also add hickory nuts for a different taste to your muffin.

### 132. Blueberry honey muffin

Aside from using bananas, you can also use candied versions of the berries available in your area. Blueberry muffin will also taste great with pecan.

### 133. Raspberry honey muffin

As you may have already guessed, there are many variations for this recipe. Raspberry is another replacement for banana.

### 134. Top with coconut cream

You can also improve the taste of your honey muffin and its variations if you add coconut cream on top of it while serving.

### 135. Serve with breakfast sausage

You can increase the protein content of this breakfast by adding meat. Add a breakfast sausage to this meal to make it tastier.

### 136. Paleo carrot cake

- 7 eggs
- 1 ½ tsp. vanilla extract
- Grated carrots (At least 1 cup)
- ½ cup coconut flour
- A pinch of salt
- 1 tsp. baking powder
- 1 tsp. ground cloves
- A pinch of baking soda
- 1 tsp. cinnamon
- 1 cup natural honey
- 1 cup olive oil
- 6 tbsp. coconut butter

**Instructions:**

1. Preheat the oven to 180 degrees Celsius. Grease the pan with oil.
2. Mix the coconut flour, baking soda, salt, cinnamon and cloves in a bowl. Stir until they are thoroughly mixed.
3. In a saucepan, melt the honey and coconut butter. Add the mixture in a bowl and add the olive oil and vanilla extract.

4. Lastly, add the grated carrots and eggs and blend them until you have a fine mixture.
5. Combine the dry ingredients and continue blending.
6. Pour the mixture to the pan and bake for 20-25 to the desired firm consistency.

Serves 6 people

### 137. Coconut-carrot muffin

You can also add grated coconut meat to the mix to add a grainy and crunchy texture to the carrot muffin. Add it when you are mixing the batter. ½ cup should be enough.

### 138. Top with blueberries

You can also top the muffins with blueberry and honey to make it sweeter.

### 139. Serve with carrot sticks and bacon

When serving your carrot muffin, you can add bulk to the meal by adding carrot sticks. You can also add a salty flavor by adding bacon.

### 140. Add sweet guacamole

You can also add guacamole sweetened by raw honey. The taste of the guacamole will contrast that of the muffin without adding too much calories.

### 141. Paleo Sweet Potato Muffins

**Ingredients:**

- 1 cup mashed sweet potato
- ¼ tsp. nutmeg
- 1 ½ tsp. baking powder

- 3 eggs
- ¼ cup honey
- 1 cup almond flour
- ¾ cup raisins
- ¾ cup grated apple
- ¾ cup shredded coconut
- ¾ cup shredded carrot
- ½ cup chopped dried figs
- ¾ cup chopped walnuts
- 1 ½ tsp. cinnamon

## Instructions:

1. Preheat the oven to 175 degrees Celsius while mixing all the ingredients in a bowl.
2. Glaze muffin pan with coconut oil andpour the batter to make nine muffins.
3. Put the muffins in the oven and let it bake for 30-40 minutes.
4. You will know that it's ready when the top is golden brown.

### 142. Cooked mashed squashes for alternative

You can also use cooked squash to replace sweet potato if you do not like the taste. Mash it and use equal amounts as suggested by the instructions. They taste different but squash adds a lot more nutrients to the dish.

### 143. Choco-Banana Paleo Pancakes

## Ingredients:

- 6medium eggs

- 3ripe bananas (mashed)
- 3 tbsp. almond butter
- ½ cup Chocolate chips (Dark)

**Instructions:**

1. Mix the mashed bananas, almond butterand eggs in a large bowl. Add half of the chocolate chips with the batter.
2. In a flat pan, pour ¼ cup of the batter to make a pancake shape. Cook it in medium heat. Flip when bubbles show in the corners.
3. Cook the other side for around one minute and a half.
4. Mix well and scoop a quarter of a cup of the mixture on to a hot griddle or flat pan over medium heat. Wait for bubbles to appear then flip and cook for another one-two minutes.
5. Sprinkle the rest of the chocolate chips before serving.

Serves 6 people

### 144. Make it more chocolatey

You can make the chocolate flavor even stronger by adding cocoa powder as you mix the batter.

### 145. Choco-Banana Paleo Pancakes Paleo withbacon

You can make the previous breakfast recipe even tastier by serving it with crispy sugar-free bacon baked in ghee.

### 146. Coconut Choco-Banana Paleo Pancakes

You can change the almond butter in the previous recipe with any nut paste. Coconut butter for example, is a great substitute to almond butter.

## 147. Strawberry coconut-banana Paleo Pancakes

If you do choose to use coconut butter, you can also remove the chocolate chips and add strawberries. Make the batter with the banana and the coconut butter and add thinly sliced strawberries when serving.

## 148. Broccoli with eggs salad paleo breakfast

**Ingredients**:

- 2 medium eggs (Cooked over easy)
- 1 tbsp. onions(chopped)
- 1 medium carrot (sliced)
- 2 large sliced thick tomatoes
- ¼ cup chopped celery
- 1 cup chopped broccoli

**Instructions:**

1. In mixing bowl, add all the ingredients except for the eggs and then toss.
2. Place the tossed vegetables in your two serving plates.
3. Once the eggs are cooked, add them on top of the salad.

Serves 2 people

## 149. Spinach with eggs salad paleo breakfast

You can easily tweak the above recipe by changing the broccoli with your choice of green leafy vegetables. For example, use green spinach.

## 150. Double green-leafy variation

You can also use both green spinach and broccoli on the same dish to even add more green leafy vegetables to your breakfast.

### 151. Arugula with eggs paleo salad

Arugula is another vegetable that you can use instead of broccoli in the egg salad. You should be aware however, that it changes the flavor of the salad. It adds a pepper and mustard-like tinge to your salad.

### 152. Green leafy paleo salad with avocadoes and eggs

You can add more flavor to your vegetable and egg salad by adding diced avocadoes to the mix when tossing it.

### 153. Romaine Lettuce with eggs paleo salad

Romaine lettuce is also an effective green leafy vegetable to add to your egg salad breakfast. You can use the avocado variation with this green leafy vegetable as well.

### 154. Escarole and lettuce with eggs paleo salad

If the taste of romaine lettuce is too sweet of a vegetable for you, you can add a bitter tinge to the egg salad by adding escarole.

### 155. Vitamin-rich Green-leafy vegetable salad

If you are in need of more dietary vitamins, you can use curly endive and escarole with broccoli to make your salad. They are both rich in Vitamins A, E, and C. Adding 2 cups of each will provide a big boost in your daily intake of these vitamins.

### 156. Watercress and broccoli salad with egg

You can also add watercress to your salad mix to make the dish more nutritious. It is rich in calcium and adding two cups will only add 8 calories to your meal.

### 157. Pecan and Greens egg breakfast salad

You can add more variety to your egg salad by adding nuts to the mix. Add chopped pecan to add a hard texture to your green-leafy salads.

### 158. Green-leafy egg salads with fruits

If you want to add sweet fruit flavors to the recipe, simply slice up an apple, a pear and some grapes. They will provide you with the sucrose you need in the morning.

### 159. Broccoli and chickpeas with eggs salad paleo breakfast

Chickpeas also work well in adding more filling to your salad. If you want to be full in your first meal, this add-on will get the job done.

### 160. Broccoli with eggs and dried apricots salad paleo breakfast

Dried fruits also work well with most salads. Your broccoli and eggs for instance will taste even sweeter with dried apricots. They also add more texture to the dish.

### 161. Romaine lettuce with eggs and dried cranberries salad paleo breakfast

Dried cranberries also work well with most green leafy salads. They are best added to the romaine lettuce version of the recipe.

### 162. Double Green leafy vegetables with mango paleo breakfast smoothie

- ¼ cup of Spinach
- ¼ cup of Kale
- 1 large Mango (pulp)
- Raw honey to taste

- Ice
- 2 hard-boiled eggs

**Instructions:**

1. Add all the ingredients except for the honey to the blender.
2. Blend until smooth. Taste the smoothie to know how much honey to add.
3. Add honey to your desired sweetness.
4. Pour the smoothie to your serving glass and serve with 2 hardboiled eggs.

### 163. Mango avocado paleo smoothie

In the recipe above, you can remove one of the green leafy vegetables and add 2 avocadoes to the mix. For example, use kale, mango and avocados for your smoothie.

### 164. Double Green leafy smoothie with raw Yacon syrup

People are still arguing with how paleo honey is. If you don't have access to naturally harvested honey, you can replace it with raw Yacon syrup. This type of sweetener has a different kind of sweetness but it still gets the job done.

### 165. African berries mango paleo smoothie

There is a big hype behind the healthiness of African berries. Though most of these claims are unverified, they are best used as a sugar substitute. You do not add this berry to your smoothie. Instead, you slice it and rub it in your tongue.

### 166. Miracle berries with avocado and spinach paleo smoothie

Normally, you wouldn't create an avocado spinach recipe without a sweetener. However, you can do it by rubbing miracle berries to your tongue. They will make the seemingly tasteless smoothie sweeter.

## 167. Low carb breakfast bar

### Ingredients:

- 4 cups of different seeds and nuts(slivered almonds, sunflower seeds,walnuts)
- 1 ½ cup dried apricot and cranberry mix
- 3 cups coconuts meat (shredded and unsweetened)
- ½ cup coconut oil
- ¾ cup almond butter
- ¾ cup raw honey
- ½ tsp. vanilla extract
- ¾ tsp. sea salt
- 1 ½ tsp. cinnamon

### Instructions:

1. Chop the larger nuts into smaller pieces.
2. In a mixing bowl, pour the nuts and seeds and mix.
3. Put half of the mixed nuts in a food processor and pulse it to make them finer.
4. Mix them back with the other nuts in the mixing bowl.
5. Add the dried fruits to the mix and the shredded coconut and stir it.
6. Prepare a small pan by adding almond butter, honey, coconut oil cinnamon and salt into it.
7. Cook the pan in medium low heat while stirring it until bubbles start to show.

8. Remove the pan and add the heated liquid to the assorted nuts and seeds. Combine them by stirring.
9. Prepare a 9x13 baking dish. Add parchment paper over it.
10. When everything is mixed well, pour the mixture on the baking dish.
11. Let it settle for one and a half hours.
12. Cover it and put it in the freezer. Use a second layer of parchment paper to cover it.
13. Cut to preferred serving size and serve.

### 168. Low carb paleo cereal

The above recipe also works well as a cereal substitute. If you want a breakfast cereal, break the bar apart with your hands and add coconut milk to it. Add honey as sweetener.

### 169. Mixed nuts bar with smoothie

You can also serve the above bar with any of the previously discussed smoothies. They can work well to add fiber bulk to your breakfast.

### 170. Mixed nuts bar with Fresh fruits

We also suggest using the mixed nuts bar with fresh fruits that are in season. Serve them with mangoes, avocadoes, apples and pears. You should then add honey over the fruits to add a sweet flavor.

### 171. Low carb paleo cereal with almond milk, bacon and smoothies

Your low carb cereal can also be served with almond milk. You should add unsweetened bacon together with your choice of smoothies to make your breakfast bigger. This nutty cereal, meat and smoothie combo should increase your caloric intake early.

### 172. Banana apple smoothies

## Ingredients:

- 4 bananas (peeled)
- 4 ripe organic apples (Core removed and sliced into four pieces each)
- 3 cups organic baby spinach (washed)
- 2Persian cucumber (washed, tips removed, cut into three chunks)
- Ice cubes
- Organic honey to taste

## Instructions:

1. Add the ingredients in the following order: Banana at the bottom, apples, cucumber, spinach and ice.
2. Blend until smooth.
3. Add the honey to taste.
4. If it is too sweet, add ice and pulse.
5. Pour in a glass and serve with 2 pieces of unsweetened bacon.

### 173. Milky Banana apple smoothies

You can add a milky variation by adding coconut milk to the smoothie recipe. The banana will taste great with the milky flavor.

### 174. Nutty Milky Banana and apple smoothie

Instead of adding coconut milk, you can use almond milk to add a nutty flavor to your smoothie. The almond milk will also enhance the taste of the banana.

### 175. Triple tropical fruit breakfast smoothie

- 4 bananas (peeled)
- 2 ripe mangoes (Seed removed and pulp sliced cubes)
- 3 cups organic baby spinach (washed)
- 2avocadoes (core removed, removed from peel, cut into cubes)
- Ice cubes
- Coconut milk
- Organic honey to taste

## Instructions:

1. Blend the ingredients as instructed in previous smoothie recipes.
2. Add coconut milk and honey to taste.

### 176. Kale variation of the tropical fruit smoothie

Aside from baby spinach, you can also use kale.

### 177. The peach variation

Peach also tastes great with the bananas and avocadoes. If the peach is too sweet, you may lessen the amount of honey to control the sweetness.

### 178. Paleo Banana-avocado smoothie

## Ingredients:

- 4 bananas (peeled)
- 2 cups organic kale (washed)
- 2avocadoes (core removed, removed from peel, cut into cubes)
- Watermelon pulp (seeds removed and cut into cubes)

- Ice cubes
- Organic honey to taste

## Instructions:

1. Do the same as with other smoothie instructions.
2. This version does not taste well with coconut or almond milk.
3. Serve with mixed nuts cereal above.

### 179. Mango-avocado smoothie

You can also use the recipe with mangoes instead of bananas. You should take advantage when this fruit is in season. It will add a sweeter taste to your smoothie, depending on the sweetness of the mangoes.

### 180. Nectarine version

You can also pair your avocados with nectarine. They also taste great in smoothies.

### 181. Peach –avocado version

If you are tired of bananas but the other fruits suggested above are not available, you can add peaches instead. They are more abundant than tropical fruits and their pulp tastes great in smoothies.

### 182. Paleo Almond Pancakes with Fresh Blueberries

## Ingredients:

- 2 cup almond flour
- 1 cup unsweetened applesauce
- 2 tbsp. coconut flour

- 4 large eggs
- 1/2 cup soda water
- 1/2 tsp. freshnutmeg
- 1/2 tsp. seasalt
- 2 tbsp. coconut oil
- 1 cup blueberries

**Instructions:**

1. In a mixing bowl, mix the almond flour, sea salt, coconut flour, applesauce, eggs, soda water, and nutmeg.
2. Grease a skillet with coconut oil in medium-low heat.
3. Pour 1/8 of the batter to the pan to make pancake shapes.
4. When bubbles begin to show at the sides and on the top, add a few berries on top before flipping. Keep it in the heat for another 1 ½ minutes.
5. Repeat the process with the rest of the batter.
6. Serve with blueberries.

Serves 4 people

### 183. Paleo Almond Pancakes with bananas and mangoes

Pancakes can be modified in many ways. This particular recipe can be tweaked a little by adding bananas and mangoes instead of berries. Add mashed banana to the batter and serve the pancakes with sliced bananas and mangoes.

### 184. Paleo Almond Pancakes with bananas and apples

Bananas also taste great with apples in the mix. Because of the applesauce, you can add apple when serving this version of a pancake.

### 185. Paleo Almond Pancakes with raspberries

You can change the blueberry in the recipe to any type of sweet berry. Follow the instructions but instead of using blueberries, you can use raspberries.

### 186. Paleo Almond Pancakes with mixed berries

Some people also choose to add both blueberries and raspberries when serving. This will add a richer flavor to your pancakes but it also raises the calories per serving.

### 187. Paleo Almond Pancakes with berries and pear

Most people never try to experiment with the fruits that they add to their pancakes. Because pancakes have a fairly neutral flavor, add more fruits like pear when serving it.

### 188. Paleo Almond Pancakes with roasted almond on the side

You will even bring out the flavor of your blueberry almond pancakes if you serve it with roasted almonds.

### 189. Nutty paleo version of an oatmeal

**Ingredients:**

- 3 cups unsweetened applesauce
- 8 tbsp. raw and chunky almond butter
- 4 tbsp. unsweetened fresh coconut milk
- 2 tsp. cinnamon, to taste
- 2 tsp. fresh and grated nutmeg
- 1 cup dried assorted nuts

**Instructions:**

1. Mix all ingredients in a bowl except for the nuts.

2. Add them to a small pan at medium heat until the mixture is warm.
3. Put the heated mixture in a serving bowl and add the dried assorted nuts.

Serves 4 people

### 190. Serve with bananas

You can add more fiber to the recipe by adding thick slices of banana over the liquid before serving it.

### 191. Add sliced avocados

If you want to add more flavors to your oatmeal, add slices of freshly sliced avocados over it. You may serve them together with the banana slices as suggested above.

### 192. Using dried fruits

If you want more variety to this recipe, use dried apricot and cranberries instead of dried seeds. This adds more texture to the recipe.

### 193. Serve it with smoothie

If you have a busy day ahead, you may also serve it with some of our smoothies in this book. This will increase the calorie content of your meal.

Add slices of fruits

This recipe has a nutty sweet flavor to it. Add a sourer flavor to it by adding some of your favorite fruits when serving it. You can add slices of apple and pear for example to add more fruits to your meal.

### 194. Arugula with fruits paleo salad

- 4 large oranges
- 2 large avocado, diced
- 1/2 cup raw cashews
- 6 cups arugula
- 2 tbsp. olive oil
- 1/2 tsp. sea salt (to taste)
- 1/4 tsp. black pepper (to taste)
- 4 chicken breast, (boneless and skinless), grilled and sliced into cubes

## Instructions:

1. Peel the orange and divide it into wedges. Remove the veins to make it clean. Slice each wedge crosswise but try to lose as little juice as possible.
2. Equally distribute the arugula to 4 plates. Add the orange, diced avocado,and cashews on top of the greens.
3. Add olive oil on top of the salad and the juice that may have spilled when slicing the orange wedges. Add the pepper and salt to taste.
4. Add the diced chicken on top of it and serve.

Serves 4 people

### 195. Watercress version

You can also make this recipe by replacing the arugula with watercress. The taste of the greens will slightly change but they still taste great with the orange and avocados.

### 196. Add more orange juice

Some people prefer to add more orange juice to make the salad wet. If this is what you want, you should leave 2 or 3 orange wedges unsliced. When adding the olive oil, squeeze these wedges over your salad to add the juice.

### 197. Baby spinach version

If spinach is more abundant in your area, you can use it to replace arugula.

### 198. Three-leaf version

If you are lucky enough to have arugula, spinach and watercress in your area, you should consider adding all of them in the mix. This will add texture and flavor to your salad.

### 199. The leafy salad without the chicken

If you want a light breakfast, remove the chicken from the recipe. The chicken added a large bulk of calories to the mix. If you remove it, you will be able to remove a large amount of calories from the recipe.

### 200. Add chopped almonds for bulk

If you want more healthy calories in your meal, you should add chopped roasted almonds to the mix. You should make sure that they are unsalted and unsweetened.

### 201. Turkey version

Grilled chicken tastes great but if you have leftover turkey during thanksgiving, you can use it to enrich this dish. Grill it and cut it into small cubes.

### 202. Coconut-lime berry breakfast

## Ingredients:

- 2 cups fresh assorted berries
- 1/2 cup fresh coconut milk
- 1 medium-sized lime

## Instructions:

1. Distributethe berries into four small bowls.
2. Add coconut milk, and mix.
3. Squeeze lime juice over it before serving.

Serves 4 people

### 203. The berries and nuts version

Assorted berries are not available all the time. If only one type of berry is available in your area, you may supplement your breakfast with unsalted assorted nuts instead.

### 204. The almond milk version

You can also use almond milk instead of coconut milk. Though coconut milk tastes better with lime juice, almond milk still tastes good. Use it to add variety to your breakfast.

### 205. The coconut-lemon version

Most citrus juice tastes good with coconut milk. Replace the lime with freshly squeezed lemon juice. You should use this version if you want your bowl to be sweeter rather than tangy.

### 206. Single Berry version

There may be times when a certain type of berry is more abundant. If this is the case, you may use just one type of berry. If there is a high supply of blueberries for example, you can use fresh blueberries for breakfast.

### 207. Serve with bacon

You can also choose to serve this with bacon fried in ghee. Some people also like breaking the bacon apart and sprinkling it in the bowl with the berries.

### 208. Eat with fruit smoothies

You may also choose to serve this dish with a glass of freshly prepared cold smoothies for hot mornings. If there is an abundance of mangoes in the season for example, you can serve mango smoothies with this dish.

### 209. Add granola bar crumbles for texture and taste

If you prefer cereals in the morning, take a granola bar, break it apart and add the pieces to the bowl of berries. This will add hard texture to your breakfast. It will also add protein.

### 210. Assorted berries bowl with avocado slices

If you want to add bulk to your bowl of assorted berries, add avocado slices to the mix. You should keep the slices small so that they will mix well with the berries.

### 211. Assorted berries bowl with tropical fruits

You should also keep yourself familiar with the available tropical fruits in the season. If there are a lot of watermelons for example, you may also choose to serve the bowl with a slice of watermelon on the side.

## 212. Assorted berries bowl with dried fruits

Dried fruits are also effective in adding texture and taste to the berry bowl. You may choose paleo fruits like apricot and cranberries. Adding this to your meal plan will add variety to your diet.

## 213. Paleo-version Granola mix

### Ingredients:

- 1/2 cup slivered almonds
- 1/2 cup chopped pecans
- 1/2 cup chopped walnuts
- 1/4 cup raw sunflower seeds
- 1/4 cup raw pumpkin seeds
- 1 tbsp. chia seeds
- 1 tbsp. ground flax seeds
- 1 tbsp. melted coconut oil
- 1/2 tbsp. raw honey
- Pinch of cinnamon
- 1/2 cup raisins
- 1/2 cup goji berries

### Instructions:

1. Preheat oven to 135 degrees Celsius.
2. In a large mixing bowl, mix the pecans, almonds, sunflower seeds, pumpkin seeds, chia, flax, walnuts, coconut oil, maple syrup and cinnamon.
3. Spread evenly in a baking pan covered with parchment paper. Bake for 18-20 minutes.

4. Remove it from the oven and let it cool. Add the raisins and the goji berries on top of it and serve warm with almond milk.

### 214. Granola mix cereal

Just like the other recipe for granola bar in this book, you can also convert this granola mix into a nutty cereal. Instead of serving it by itself, break it apart and serve it in a bowl of cold or warm coconut milk.

### 215. Granola cereal and berries

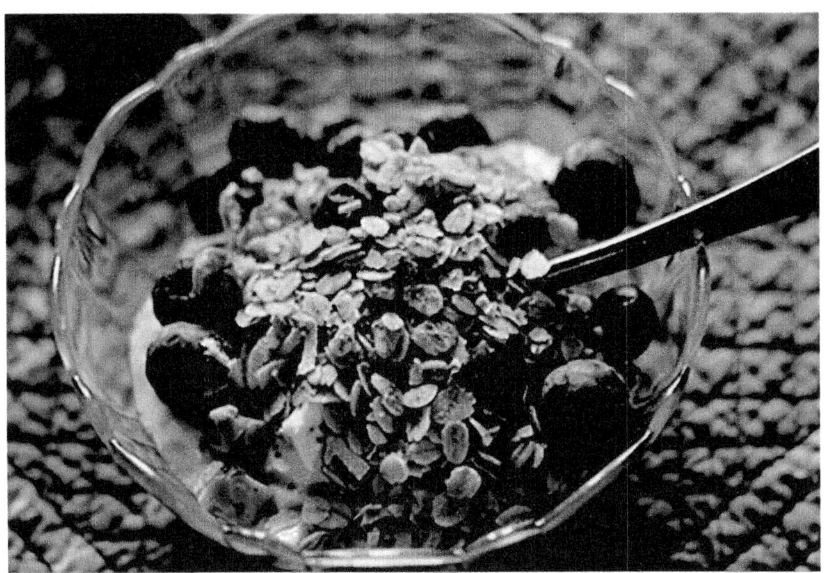

**Photo Source: https://pixabay.com/en/breakfast-yogurt-healthy-352461/**

You can also add berries to your nutty granola cereal. Use chilled coconut milk to make it refreshing in the morning. You should then add fresh blueberries, raspberries and sliced strawberries.

### 216. Granola cereal and dried fruits

You can also add more natural sweetness to your granola cereal by adding dried apricots and cranberries to it. The concentrated taste of these dried fruits will explode in your mouth. It also gives you something to bite into.

### 217. Granola cereal and avocado slices

If you are using chilled coconut milk, add slices of peeled and pitted avocadoes to go with the granola mix cereal. The softer avocado will add more texture to the cereal bowl.

### 218. Serve with fresh fruits

The granola bar will taste dry if you eat it by itself. If you want to add moisture to your breakfast, serve it with fresh ripe papaya or pear slices.

### 219. Kiwi and Strawberry Breakfast Smoothie

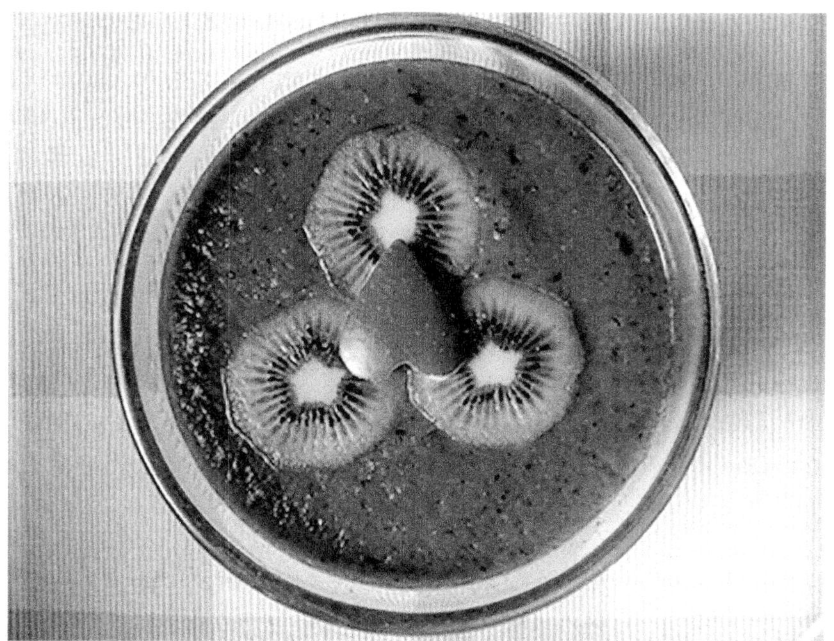

**Photo Source: https://pixabay.com/en/smoothie-nutrition-drink-bio-1166399/**

**Ingredients:**

- 2 large peeled and roughly sliced kiwis
- 2 cups frozen strawberries
- 2 cans coconut milk
- 4 tbsp. chia seeds
- 2 tsp. raw honey

**Instructions:**

1. Pulse the kiwi, strawberries, coconut milk and honey for 45 seconds.
2. Put the mixture in cups and add the chia seeds.

Serves 4 people

### 220. Serve with bacon and other breakfast meat

Though the smoothie can be a standalone meal, you may also add a salty taste to your meals by serving it with breakfast meats like bacon and ham.

### 221. The chunky variation

Some people like to have something to bite into when taking their smoothies for breakfast. If you prefer your fruit smoothie with chunky bits of fruit, you should divide the strawberries into two. You should pulse the first half with the mixture for 30 seconds. You should then add the next batch and pulse it at low power for only 10 seconds.

### 222. Kiwi, strawberries and lime juice smoothie

Lime juice makes all sweet drinks more interesting. The coconut milk in your kiwi and strawberry smoothie will taste even better if you enhance it with lime juice.

## 223. Kiwi, strawberry and mango version

You can also try adding mangoes to this smoothie when it is in season. To prevent the mangoes from overpowering the taste of the smoothie, you should limit the amount that you add. Use half a tablespoon of mashed pulp for each serving.

## 224. Vegetable Pizza Frittata breakfast

### Ingredients:

- 5 eggs
- 1 ½ tbsp. dry chopped basil
- ½ tbsp. dry chopped oregano
- ½ kg tomato puree
- 3 crushed garlic cloves
- Nutritional yeast
- 1 tbsp. olive oil
- 1 tsp. salt
- 1 medium zucchini (sliced lengthwise)

### Instructions:

1. Preheat oven to 180 degrees Celsius.
2. In a bowl, crack the eggs and whisk.Add the rest of ingredients except for zucchini. Mix them all.
3. Pour a third of the egg-tomato mixture (1 ¼ cup) into 9x13 inch pan. Make sure that you cover the bottom.
4. Arrange the zucchini slices on the pan, similar to how you would line a pan when cooking lasagna.
5. Cover the zucchini layer with 1/3 of egg mixture. Add another layer of zucchini, and top with the rest of the egg mixture.

6. Bake the pan for 45 minutes. You will know that it's cooked when the top is red.
7. Remove from the oven and cut it into squares before serving.

### 225. Meaty vegetable frittatas

You can add meat of your choice to this dish if you want. Use boiled and shredded chicken breasts. You can also use shredded turkey meat. You should add them to the mixture in step b.

### 226. Zucchini frittata muffins

Instead of using a regular frittata dish, you can convert this dish into a frittata muffin by placing the mixture in muffin tins glazed with coconut oil. This version is easier to carry and works better for people who bring their breakfast to work.

### 227. Serve with bacon strips

If you want a meaty flavor with this dish, you can serve bacon strips along with it. Use turkey bacon to limit the calorie count.

### 228. Turn it to a meaty pizza by adding ground beef on top

You can instantly add a meaty flavor to this dish by adding ground beef cooked in its own fat. You can also add mushrooms to make it seem like a real pizza.

# Chapter 6

# Paleo Breakfast Meat Recipes

**229. Paleo Ham wraps**

**Ingredients:**

- 1 medium seeded honeydew melon or melon
- 2 packages sliced ham, prosciutto
- 4 tbsp. fresh and chopped mint

**Instructions:**

1. Slice cantaloupe into 1 ½-inch wedges. Remove the rinds.
2. Use the prosciuttos to wrap the cantaloupe wedges. Use a toothpick to secure the wrap.
3. Add fresh mint as garnish. Put it in the fridge and serve cold.

Serves 8 people

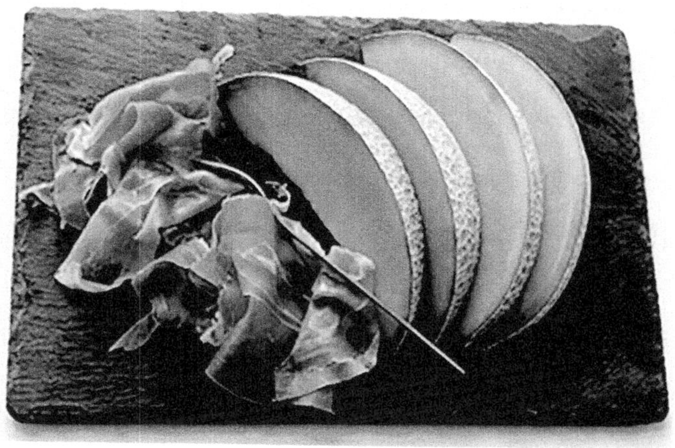

### 230. Replace honeydew with ripe papaya

The ham will also taste great with the sweetness of papaya. Slice them small and wrap them in prosciutto wraps.

### 231. Replace the fruit with cantaloupes

On hot days, you may also replace the honeydewwith cantaloupes. They are both sweet. They are a very good alternative if honeydew is not available in your area.

### 232. Make them with smoothies on the run

You can prepare this type of breakfast easily. If you are in a hurry, prepare a decent number of ham wrapped fruits before leaving your home. You can then take them with you on the road.

### 233. Bacon wrapped fruits

**Ingredients:**

- 4 slices bacon
- 8 medium Medjool dates
- 8 medium whole almonds

**Instructions:**

1. Open dates with a knife.
2. Put a whole almond inside each date.
3. Wrap it with the bacon. Slice the bacon in half if needed.
4. Preheat the oven at 190 degrees Celsius.
5. Place on a baking sheet and bake the bacon for about 6 minutes.
6. Flip the bacon and bake until bacon is crispy.
7. Serve warm with smoothie of choice.

### 234. Replace bacon with ham slices

You can also choose to replace bacon with ham slices. They will not be as crispy but they will add a different flavor.

### 235. Serve with fresh papaya slices

The breakfast finger foods will taste salty and sweet at the same time. However, on its own, the bacon-wrapped dates will seem dry. To add more moisture to the dish, you may add fresh fruit slices. This will also add bulk to your meal.

### 236. Smoothie and bacon-wrapped dates

You can also add moisture to the breakfast dish by consuming it with some of the paleo smoothies discussed in this book.

### 237. Berries and nuts with coconut and lime mix

## Ingredients:

- 2 cups strawberries, blueberries, raspberries
- 2 cups assorted unsalted nuts
- 1/2 cupcoconut milk
- 1 medium orange

## Instructions:

1. Slice the berries and chop the nuts.
2. Add them to your mixing bowl and mix.
3. Add the orange juice last and mix thoroughly.

### 238. Fruits alternative to berries

There are also varieties of foods that you can replace the berries with. For instance, you can use 2 cups of sliced watermelon, cantaloupes, and papaya. If you want bigger slices of these fruits, you should add the amount of orange juice use.

### 239. Use almonds instead of nuts

You can also replace the nuts with almonds. Use slivered ones to keel the size small. You should make sure that you don't use those salted brands.

### 240. Paleo Ham Wrapped Frittata muffins

- 8tbsp. coconut oil
- 1 medium diced onion
- 6 cloves of garlic(minced)
- ½ kg. thinly slicedcremini mushrooms
- ½ kg. spinach
- ½ cup coconut milk
- 4tbsp. of coconut flour
- 16 large eggs
- 2 cups halved cherry tomatoes
- 280 grams Prosciutto
- Freshly ground pepper to taste
- Kosher salt to taste
- 2 regular 12 cup muffin tin

## Instructions:

1. Preheat the oven to 190°C and prepare the veggies.
2. Over medium heat, heat half of the coconut oil in a large cast iron skillet. Sauté the onions until they are soft.
3. Add the garlic and mushrooms and cook them until the moisture has evaporated off the mushrooms. Season the filling with salt and pepper. Transfer it to a plate and let it cool.

4. Beat the eggs in a large bowl with salt, coconut flour, coconut milk and pepper until well mixed. Add the sautéed spinach and mushroom. Stir them to mix.
5. Brush the coconut oil into the muffin tin. Line each cup with prosciutto. You should make sure tocover the entire bottom and sides.
6. Spoon the frittata batter into them and top each muffin cups with halved cherry tomatoes.
7. Bake the batch for 20 minutes. Rotate the tray after 10 minutes.

Serves 8 people

### 241. Kosher pastrami substitute for the ham

Prosciutto is difficult to replace if it is not available. However, if this is the case, you should try kosher pastrami from your local store.

### 242. Arugula as a spinach alternative

Spinach is another difficult ingredient to replace. However, if you do not mind the added mustard-like flavor, you can use arugula in its place.

### 243. Using baby lettuce for spinach

Baby lettuce may also work as alternative to the vegetable. It may not be as tasty but it will be effective in replacing the spinach if the latter is not available.

### 244. Serve with guacamole

The guacamole's taste will contrast with that of the frittata muffin, which will enrich the whole experience.

### 245. Try with avocado-based smoothies

If you like smoothies better than guacamole, try the ones with avocadoes. The taste of avocadoes will lessen the salty taste of the ham.

### 246. Serve with paleo coleslaw

The salty taste of the ham wrapped frittata will also blend well with paleo coleslaw with mild vinaigrette, cabbage, red onions and carrots.

### 247. Serve with green leafy salads

You can also blend the flavors of this frittata with the green salads. A simple bowl of vinaigrette, raw spinach and tomatoes will blend well with this dish.

### 248. Spicy bacon frittata

## Ingredients:

- 2 tbsp. coconut oil for sautéing
- 1 tsp. coconut oil for greasing
- 12smoked organic diced bacon
- 12-15diced button mushrooms
- 2 deseeded and chopped jalapeno peppers
- 12 large eggs
- 1 cup coconut milk (Full fat)
- Salt and pepper, to taste

## Instructions:

1. Preheat the oven to180 degrees Celsius. Use coconut oil to grease an 8 inch round pie baking tin.

2. In medium heat, heat 1 tablespoon of coconut oil in a skillet. Add the bacon, mushrooms and jalapenos. Sauté the ingredients for 2 minutes. By the end of the second minute, the bacon should begin to become crispy.
3. Crack the eggs into a large mixing bowl and whisk. Add the coconut milk until the mixture becomes light and air bubbles appear.
4. Add the sautéed mushroom, bacon and jalapenos to the mixing bowl, and add salt and pepper to taste. Distribute the frittata mixture into the pie tin.
5. Bake for 20-30 minutes. Check if the middle is cooked with a toothpick.

### 249. The turkey strips alternative

If you want to use less fatty types of meats, you can use strips of turkey meat or even turkey bacon. The taste is not as strong as the real bacon but it is a healthier alternative.

### 250. Spicy bacon frittata muffins

You can also convert this dish into a frittata muffin by baking it in muffin tins. You should make sure however, that you glaze the muffin tin with coconut oil so that the frittatas do not stick.

### 251. Serve with grilled vegetables

The spicy taste of the frittata will lessen if you serve it with grilled bell pepper and tomatoes.

### 252. Serve with guacamole to make it less spicy

If the frittata turned out to be too spicy, serve it with guacamole to lessen the heat. You may also serve it with fruit smoothies.

## 253. Chicken and bacon frittata

- 1 large Onion(chopped)
- 2 cooked and shredded Chicken breasts
- 10 bacon strips(cooked and chopped)
- 15 large Eggs
- 1/2 tsp. Sea salt
- ½ cup full-fat Coconut milk
- 2 tbsp. Coconut oil
- 1/4 tsp. Garlic powder
- 1 Tomato medium in size and slicedthinly
- Freshly cracked Pepper to taste
- Coconut oil mix:
- 4 tbsp. Coconut oil
- 1 tsp. Garlic(minced)
- 1 scallion (minced)
- A small squeeze of lemon juice

## Instructions:

1. Preheat oven to 200 degrees.
2. In a cast iron skillet over medium fire, heat coconut oil until it is shimmering. Add the onion then start to sauté for about 3 and a half minutes.
3. In a bowl, whisk the coconut milk, eggs, salt and pepper. Add the chicken and bacon to the skillet.
4. Pour the ranch over the top, stir to combine.
5. Evenly spread the mixture on the skillet.Place the eggs on the top.
6. Evenly arrange the tomato slices on the top.

7. Sprinkle garlic powder on top of it and add more chopped bacon.
8. Let it cook for 4 minutes or until the edges are starting to lift.
9. Transfer it to the oven and cook for 12 minutes.
10. After baking, let it cool. Once cool, use a knife to separate the edges from the baking skillet.
11. Keep it refrigerated until serving day. Reheat before serving.

Serves 7-8 people

### 254. Chicken and bacon frittata muffins

You can also convert this dish and any of its variations into meat muffins by cooking them in muffin tins. You can use the instructions above, but instead of using an oven-ready skillet, you should use a muffin tin when baking them.

### 255. Turkey bacon variation

You may also use turkey bacon in this recipe to lessen the fat content of your breakfast.

### 256. Macon and chicken also tastes great

You can also use Macon instead of bacon. The meat duo also tastes great in the frittata mixture.

### 257. Replace chicken with turkey meat

Chicken meat is more abundant but turkey meat is tastier. After thanksgiving, if you have an oversupply of turkey, you may choose to use it in the dish instead of regular chicken.

## 258. Spicy salmon frittata

### Ingredients:

- 2tbsp. coconut oil
- 2 green peppers
- 2 onions
- 4 garlic cloves
- 3 cups cherry tomatoes
- 2 tsp. cumin
- 1 tsp. paprika
- Pepper and sea salt(to taste)
- 12 eggs
- 1 cup wild salmon (you can use canned)
- 2 tbsp. chopped cilantro

### Instructions:

1. Preheat the oven to 177 degrees Celsius.
2. Beat the eggs.
3. Mince the garlic.
4. Chop the onions and peppers.
5. Using medium heat, melt the coconut oil in a skillet.
6. Sautee the chopped onions and peppers for a couple of minutes. Add the garlic last. As you stir, add the paprika, salt, pepper and cumin. Then addthe halved tomatoes when all the other veggies are cooked.
7. Add the salmon when the tomatoes are soften. Cover the entire content of the skillet in eggs.
8. Taste the content of the skillet, add salt, and pepper if necessary.

9. Transfer the contents of the pan an oven safe container without disturbing the layers. Bake for 15 minutes.
10. Remove the frittata from the oven and add cilantro before serving.

Serves 8 people

### 259. Spicy salmon frittata muffins

If you have kids, they will enjoy this breakfast dish even more if you prepare it in muffin tins. The frittatas will take the shape of the muffin tins. They will be like small meat pies for breakfast.

### 260. Tuna alternative to salmon

Though salmon is difficult to replace, you can use tuna in its place if you don't find any salmon in the market. The tuna will also taste great with the spicy tinge.

### 261. Paleo Turkey Meatball Breakfast

**Ingredients:**

- 1kg. ground turkey
- 3 eggs
- 2chopped red bell pepper
- 1 chopped small green bell pepper
- 1chopped medium sized purple onion
- 4finely diced garlic cloves
- ½ cup almond flour
- 2 tsp. sea salt
- 2 tsp. black pepper
- 2tsp. dried parsley
- 1-2 tsp. Coconut oil

**Instructions:**

1. Heat the coconut oil in a skillet under medium heat.
2. Add onions and cook for 3 minutes.
3. Add and cook the red and green bell peppers the skillet for about 2 and a half minutes. Next, add the garlic and sauté for another 3 minutes.
4. Pour the contents of the skillet to a mixing bowl. Let it standby until it's cool.
5. In another bowl, mix the turkey, salt,eggs, almond flour, andblack pepper.
6. When the sautéed ingredients have cooled, add them to the second mixing bowl.

**Making the meatballs**

1. Find some parchment paper and line your counter with it.
2. Take a handful of your mixture and form meatballs with your hands. Convert the entire mixture into meatballs.
3. In a skillet, melt coconut oil under medium heat. Fry the meatballs in the skillet while covered with a lid. Let each batch of meatball cook for 4 minutes.
4. After that time, the meatballs should be ready to be flipped. Use tongs to do it. The bottom of the meatballs should be cooked. Return the cover of the skillet if all meatballs have been flipped. The other side should take another 3-4 minutes.

Serves 6 people

### 262. Serve with cauliflower

You can serve the meatballs by themselves or accompany them with cauliflower to add greens to your diet.

### 263. Serve with steamed vegetables

You should also consider serving the dish with steamed vegetables like broccoli, carrots and green peas. Corn may also work but it adds a large amount of carbs to your meal.

### 264. Serve with parsnip mash

These meatballs also tastes great dipped in parsnip mash. Prepare them ahead of time to lessen your preparation time.

### 265. Serve with granola mix cereal

This meatball is another tasty addition to the granola cereal recipes discussed in the earlier parts of the book.

### 266. Make it spicy with paprika

If you prefer spicy meat, you can also add paprika to the meat mix. You should mix it thoroughly to make sure not paprika balls remain in the mix.

### 267. Serve with a simple bowl of leafy green salad

Meatballs taste great with simple green salads. Mix lettuce, tomatoes, red onions and almonds and toss them with vinaigrette.

### 268. Bacon and blueberry meatball

## Ingredients:

- 2 tbsp. coconut oil
- 8 slices bacon
- 1peeled and minced small piece of ginger

- 1minced medium onion
- 2 tbsp. minced cilantro
- 2 cups fresh blueberries
- 2 lbs. ground beef
- ½ tsp. crushed red pepper flakes
- 1 tbsp. balsamic vinegar
- Sea salt and ground black pepper, to taste

**Instructions:**

1. Preheat the oven to 190 degrees Celsius.
2. Use aluminum foil to line your baking sheet. Melt the coconut oil in a small skillet.Use a brush to grease the foil with the melted coconut oil.
3. Using medium heat, cook the bacon in a skillet until it is crispy. Use a paper towel afterwards to absorb the oil as you set it aside for later.
4. Add theminced ginger, onion, and cilantro to a large mixing bowl.
5. Using a food processor, pulse the blueberries. Use 1-second bursts 7-8 times on it. Add the pulsed berries to the mixing bowl.
6. Add thecrushed red pepper flakes, ground meat, salt, pepper and balsamic vinegar. Break the bacon slices apartuse it to top the contents of the mixing bowl.
7. Use your fingers to mix all ingredients.
8. Create meatball using your hands. Arrange them in the baking sheet if you are done.
9. Bake the meatballs for 15 minutes. Rotate the pan at the 7$^{th}$ minute.

10. Remove it from the oven after the time and serve hot.

Serves 6 people

### 269. Vegetarian bacon variation

If you want to turn this breakfast dish into a vegetarian meal, you can replace the bacon with vegetarian bacon.

### 270. Top with poached eggs

If you are skilled in making unbroken poached eggs, you can add on top of each meatball. If you do this, you should only serve 1 or 2 meatballs per person.

### 271. Turkey bacon also tastes great

If you want a different taste to this recipe, you can also use turkey bacon as an alternative. The texture is almost the same as real bacon but there is a slight difference in flavor.

### 272. Macon and blueberry

Aside from turkey bacon, Macon is another low fat alternative for bacon. The taste is similar to bacon but its fat layer is not as thick.

### 273. Serve with guacamole

Just like the other meatballs, this recipe can be tasty with a sweet and meaty flavor. The neutral taste of guacamole will blend well with these flavors.

### 274. Apple cinnamon meatballs

## Instructions:

- 1kg. ground turkey
- 2 cups mashed crockpot apples
- ½ cup almond flour

- 1 cup ground flaxseed
- 1 tbsp. salt
- 1 tsp. cinnamon

**Instructions:**

1. Add 3 chopped apples in a crackpot and cook until soft. Let it cool.
2. Once cool, mash the apple with a spoon. You will use 1 cup of the mashed sauce for the recipe.
3. Preheat the oven to 175 degrees Celsius.
4. Place ground meat in a mixing bowl. Add the flaxseed, apples, almond flour,cinnamon and salt. Mix them thoroughly.
5. Make the meatballs with the contents of the mixture. Arrange them in rows in a pan greased with coconut oil.
6. Bake it between 25-30 minutes.

### 275. Replace apples with pear

You can also use pear instead of apples. Though the taste will not be the same, it will leave the same texture compared to apples.

### 276. Ground beef variety

If you don't mind the added fat content, replace the ground turkey with ground beef for a tastier version of the dish.

### 277. Apple cinnamon meatballs topped with poached eggs

You can top this meatball with poached eggs to add more protein and fat to your breakfast. This simple addition will provide you with energy to start your day.

### 278. The applesauce version

If crockpot apples are not available, replace them with applesauce. The liquid however, will not be able to replace the small solids in your dish provided by the small apples.

### 279. The cashew flour version

You may also use cashew flour for this recipe instead of using almond flour.

### 280. Serve with salsa

The dish tastes great on its own but serving it with salsa enhances the flavor of the meat.

### 281. Serve with scrambled eggs

The turkey will taste even better if you serve this dish with scrambled eggs. It will also add protein to your meal.

### 282. Serve with carrot sticks

The sweet and meaty flavors may overwhelm some people. You should give them the option to enjoy this dish with carrot sticks. This will also add more nutrients to the meal.

### 283. Serve with a bowl of lettuce, olives and tomatoes

This dish will taste great along with lettuce, olives and tomatoes garnished with vinaigrette. Choose the less sweet vinaigrette to contrast with the flavor of the meatball.

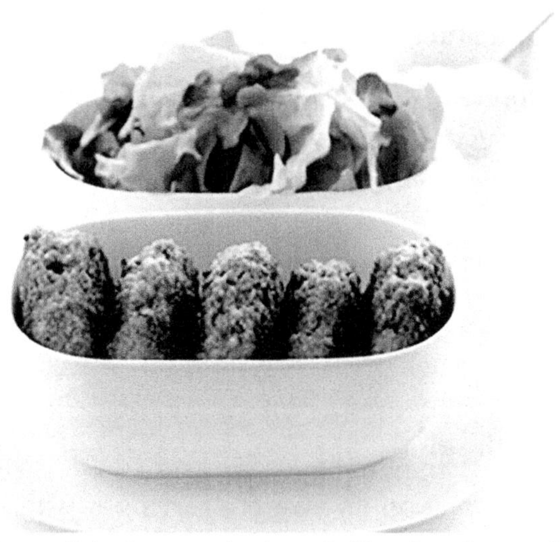

**Photo Source: https://pixabay.com/en/meatballs-minced-meat-fried-338292/**

## 284. Citrus Turkey Meatball

### Ingredients

- 500grams ground turkey
- 1 egg
- 2 diced celery stalks
- 1diced garlic cloves
- 1diced yellow onion
- ¼ cup dried cranberries
- ½ tbsp. herbs de Provence
- ½ tbsp. olive oil
- Salt and pepper to taste
- Coconut oil for greasing

### Instructions

1. Preheat oven to 200 degrees Celsius.
2. In medium heat, add olive oil, onions and celery into a skillet. Add a pinch of salt and pepper. Stir the vegetables.

After a minute, add garlic and continue sautéing.Only stop when the garlic is brown.

3. Break the dried cranberries using a knife.
4. Add the cranberries and herbs de Provence to the mix. Sautee for another 3 minutes and remove from the flame.
5. In a bowl, mix ground turkey, cooled veggie mixture and eggs. Use your hands to make meatballs. Arrange the meatballs in pan glazed with coconut oil.
6. Bake meatballs at 200 degrees Celsius for 8 minutes. Turn the pan in the oven and give it another 8 minutes or until it is fully cooked.

Serves 4 people

### 285. Citrus ground beef variation

You can also cook this dish using ground beef if ground turkey is not available.

### 286. Serve with sautéed vegetable

These meatballs will also taste better if you serve them with sautéed mixed vegetables. You can use low carb plants like broccoli, peas and carrots.

### 287. Citrus Turkey meatballs with salsa

You can also eat the turkey meatballs with salsa. You can use the salsa as a dipping sauce or you can top the meatballs with it when serving. Either way, they will taste great.

### 288. Serve with scrambled eggs and smoothies

If you want an energy packed breakfast, you should serve this breakfast meatball with unsalted scrambled eggs and smoothies.

The meatball provides the salty flavor while it is neutralized by the scrambled eggs.

### 289. Serve with green leafy salads

Meatballs also go well with green leafy salads. You can choose a salad recipe from this book.

### 290. The spicy meatball version

You can also make a spicy version by adding paprika to the meat mixture before forming the meatballs.

### 291. Paleo Turkey Breakfast Sausage

**Ingredients:**

- 1 kg.ground turkey
- 4tsp. fresh sage
- 2tsp. fresh thyme
- 2 tsp. fresh rosemary
- 1tsp. garlic powder
- 1tsp. cinnamon
- 4tbsp. coconut oil
- 2tsp. sea salt

**Instructions:**

1. Mix all the ingredients except for the oil.
2. Refrigerate for a full night.
3. Add the oil to the mixture and form patties with your hands.
4. Add more coconut oil to the skillet and cook the patties with medium heat.
5. Cook until the middle of the patty is no longer pink.

### 292. The baked variation

If you want the sausage to have a uniform consistency and crispness, you should bake it for 25 minutes at 200 degrees Celsius.

### 293. The pork version

You can also use the same recipe with organic ground pork. It will have more fat content. Use it if you are craving for the flavor of pork.

### 294. The chicken version

If turkey is not available, chicken is a better alternative because it is closest to turkey in texture. You should choose organic ground chicken with skin.

### 295. Add carrot for more vitamins

If you are planning to eat the sausages after cooking, you can also add diced carrots to the mix. The carrots will add volume and vitamins to the sausages.

### 296. Add cut-up mushrooms for flavor

Before serving it, you can also add a mushroom of your choice. You should cut them up to small pieces and add them to the mix.

### 297. Serve with caramelized onions with mushrooms

You can also add the mushrooms only when serving with caramelized onion. Sauté the mushrooms and onions while you wait for the sausages to fry.

### 298. Serve as a sausage sandwich

You can also use this recipe to make patties for your sausage sandwich. Prepare the coleslaw with cabbages, onions and carrots. Use low carb whole wheat bread for your sandwich.

### 299. Mutton sausage patty

If you have some leftover mutton lying around, you can also use that as an alternative to your turkey. They are both high in protein and low in fat.

### 300. Serve with avocado guacamole

You can make a simple avocado guacamole by mixing mashed avocado with lime juice, and chopped scallions. You should then add salt and pepper for seasoning. It will taste great with this breakfast sausage.

### 301. Add this sausage to your simple recipes

Simple recipes like scrambled eggs and green leafy salads will taste great when paired with this sausage. Slice the cooked sausage up before adding them to the other recipes.

### 302. Paleo Pork Breakfast Sausage

## Ingredients:

- 1 kg. Ground Pork
- ½ tsp. Cayenne Pepper
- ½ tsp. White Pepper
- 1 tsp. Black Pepper
- 1 tsp. Sage
- 1 tsp. Salt
- 2 tsp. Garlic
- 2 tsp. Fennel

- 2 tsp. Paprika
- 4tbsp. Organic Coconut Oil

## Instructions:

1. Mix garlic, all the spices and pork in a mixing bowl.Mix these ingredients.
2. Create 2-ounce patties from the mixture with your hands.
3. In a skillet, add the coconut oil in medium heat. Use approximately 1 tablespoon of oil per 4 patties.
4. Cook the patties until they are golden brown.

Serves 4-6 people

### 303. Spicy variation

If you want this variation to be spicier, you can add chili powder to the mix. You can also add more paprika chopped into small pieces.

### 304. Garlic heavy variation

Some people enjoy their sausages with a strong garlic flavor. You should add more chopped garlic if you prefer this flavor.

### 305. Sweet turkey breakfast sausage

You can also add a strong sweet flavor to your breakfast sausage by adding honey when mixing it.

### 306. Pork breakfast sausage with scrambled eggs

You can also serve this sausage with a generous serving of scrambled eggs. You may use some of the recipes for scrambled eggs suggested in this book.

### 307. Pork breakfast sausage with fried eggs

If you prefer fried eggs, you can have it with this pork breakfast sausage. You should use ghee or coconut oil to fry it.

### 308. Pork breakfast sausage with hard boiled eggs

The simplest way to prepare this dish is by serving it with hard-boiled eggs. The dish may seem dry so you may want to add some fruits.

### 309. Serve with fruit pancakes

The meaty flavor will complement sweet pancakes very well. You should pair them in your breakfasts.

### 310. Serve with grilled vegetables

Breakfast sausages taste great but their taste can be overpowering. Minimize the salty flavor by serving it with grilled vegetables like bell pepper, tomatoes and Brussels sprouts.

### 311. Pork breakfast sausage with steamed vegetables

Though grilled vegetables taste great, you should also consider serving it with steamed vegetables if you want a moist side dish.

### 312. Top the sausage with coleslaw

You can also use olive oil mayo to create coleslaw and put it on top of the breakfast sausage when serving.

### 313. Paleo Beef Sausage

## Ingredients:

- 6 tsp.paprika
- 4 tsp. mince garlic cloves
- 1 tsp.ground fennel seed
- 1 tsp. black pepper

- 2 tsp. sea salt
- ½ tsp.red pepper flakes
- 1 kg.groundbeef
- Coconut oil for frying

**Instructions:**

1. Combine spices in a mixing bowl.
2. Add meat and mix until all the spices are evenly distributed.
3. Form circular patties with your hands.
4. In a skillet, add the coconut oil in medium heat.
5. Cook the patties on each sideuntil the middle is no longer pink.
6. Freeze the patties if they are not yet ready to be used.
7. Reheat with ghee or coconut oil in stove for 3 minutes before serving.

Serves 4-6 people

### 314. Paleo beef breakfast sausage with grilled vegetables

You can add bulk to your beef breakfast sausage by adding grilled vegetables with it when serving. Place fresh tomatoes, bell peppers and Brussel sprouts on a stick. You should then grill them until some of the outer layers are cooked. You should then remove them from the stick and serve them with the breakfast sausage.

### 315. Serve with fresh fruits

You will need a lot of natural sugar early in the morning. For this reason, you need to add sweet fruits to your breakfast recipes. Choose watermelon, mangoes, bananas and melon. Slice them up and serve them with the breakfast sausage.

### 316. Paleo beef breakfast sausage with vegetables and eggs

You can also sauté halved tomatoes, Brussel sprouts, and spinach in a skillet over low heat. When they are done, you should add 3 eggs and let the eggs cook for a minute or so. Add it to your breakfast sausage before serving.

### 317. Paleo simple fruit smoothie with breakfast sausages

You can also serve a fruit smoothie with your breakfast sausage. You can do this by blending bananas, avocados, coconut, linseed, and almond milk. If it's a warm day, you should also add crushed ice.

### 318. Serve with granola cereal

You can also use the paleo beef breakfast sausage to add flavor to your granola cereal recipe in this book. The salty sausage will taste better if there is something sweet to contrast the taste.

### 319. Spicy paleo beef breakfast sausage

You can also add chopped paprika to the mixture if you want to give a spicy kick to the sausage. Don't overdo the paprika or the sausage may become inedible.

### 320. Sweet and spicy paleo beef breakfast sausage

If you want your pork breakfast sausage to have a sweet and spicy flavor, you can also add more natural chili powder together with honey to the mix.

### 321. Hard boiled eggs with paleo sausage

You can also serve the pork paleo sausage with your desired number of hard boiled eggs. You should make sure that the eggs are organic.

### 322. Paleo sausage with caramelized onion and mushroom

You can also sauté some onions and mushrooms to add to the breakfast sausage dish.

### 323. Paleo Taco Burger Breakfast

## Ingredients:

- 2 kg. ground chicken breast
- 1 small packet taco seasoning mix
- 2large deseeded and diced jalapeño
- 1 cup fresh chopped cilantro
- 4 tbsp. coconut oil
- 3 ripe peeled and pitted avocados
- 4 freshly squeezedlime juice
- 6 finely chopped scallions
- Salt and pepper to taste

## Instructions:

1. Mix the chicken, jalapeno, cilantro and taco seasoning in a mixing bowl.
2. Use your hands to make patties.
3. In a skillet, melt the coconut oil under low heat.
4. Cook the patties in the skillet until the middle is brown and crisp.
5. While cooking the chicken, mash the avocadoes, lime juice, and scallions. Season with salt and pepper.
6. Serve the chicken patties with the guacamole mix.

### 324. Serve with salsa

If you are fond of salsa, replace the guacamole mix with it.

### 325. Serve with grilled vegetables

You may also add grilled vegetables to the chicken and guacamole mix to add more fiber to the meal.

### 326. Add scrambled eggs

You may also use some of the scrambled egg recipes in this book and serve them with this recipe. You may even serve it with regular paleo scrambled eggs. Adding scrambled eggs will significantly increase the protein content of your dish.

### 327. Serve with fresh fruits

You may also find a seasonal fruit to serve with your burger. You can serve it with sliced papaya for example.

### 328. Prepare with avocado based drinks

This dish will also taste great with an avocado based drink. A simple avocado, coconut meat and coconut milk smoothie will significantly improve your breakfast experience.

### 329. Serve with green leafy salads

We have a few green leafy salad recipes and their variations in this book. You may use one of them to go with this dish. The neutral flavors of green leafy vegetables like lettuce and spinach will neutralize the strong taste of the meat.

### 330. Replace chicken with turkey

Ground turkey meat is an excellent substitute for chicken. Choose the lean parts and avoid adding the skin. Only add the skin if you don’t have any problems with higher fat content.

### 331. For a spicier variation, add more jalapenos

Other people like their breakfasts spicy. If you feel the same, you should add more jalapenos than suggested.

### 332. Bacon wrapped broccoli breakfast

## Ingredients:

- 2 cups slicedbroccoli leaf heads
- 1cup ghee
- 1 tbsp. paprika
- 2 tsp. onion powder
- 1 tsp. minced garlic
- 1 tsp. red pepper flakes
- 12 slices peppered bacon
- 1freshly squeezed lemon juice

## Instructions:

1. Preheat the oven at 200 degrees Celsius and prepare a baking sheet lined with parchment paper.
2. Combine garlic, onion, paprika and red pepper flakes in a bowl. When they are thoroughly mix, add the melted ghee.
3. Take a small chopped broccoli head and grease it with ghee, then dip it in the spice mixture. Do the same with the rest of the broccoli.
4. Cut the bacon in thin long strips. Wrap the broccoli heads with bacon. Use a toothpick to secure the wrap.
5. Arrange all of the wrapped broccolis in the baking sheet. Bake for 23-25 minutes.
6. Let it cool. Squeeze lemon juice over it before serving.

### 333. Serve with avocado mix

You can also use a dip made of honey, ripe avocados, lemon juice and almond milk. Blend these ingredients together until they are pasty and serve with the wrapped broccoli.

### 334. Replace Broccoli with cauliflower

You can also use cauliflower to replace the broccoli for variety.

### 335. Serve with paleo coleslaw

This salty and spicy dish can be neutralized with paleo coleslaw with red onions, cabbage and carrots.

### 336. Use guacamole

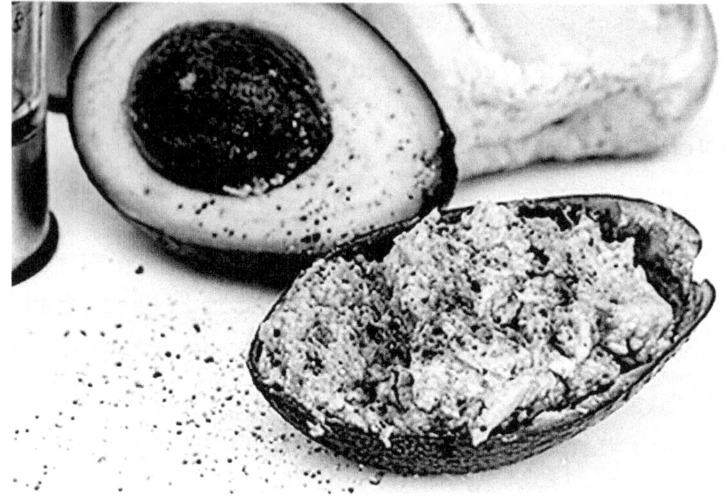

**Photo Source: https://pixabay.com/en/avocado-salad-fresh-food-829092/**

You can also use the avocado guacamole from the Paleo Taco Burger Breakfast recipe as a dip for the bacon wrapped broccoli.

### 337. Add unsalted scrambled eggs

You may also add more bulk to this recipe by adding plain, unsalted scrambled eggs on the side. The baked bacon may have a strong taste and you may want to neutralize it with eggs.

### 338. Add more paprika to make it spicier

If you are serving it with other breakfast dishes, you may want to increase the flavor of the spices. You can use paprika to add spice to the dish.

### 339. Serve with pancakes

You may use some of our pancake variations in this book to serve withthis dish. You should hold back on the dips suggested in the variation above.

### 340. Take the sweet flavor from smoothies

As with other dry foods in this recipe book, we suggest that you serve this dish with smoothies. You should avoid adding too much sweeteners in the dip.

### 341. Bacon wrapped chicken

## Ingredients:

- 2 chicken breasts
- 4slices unsweetened bacon
- 1 tbsp. olive oil

## Instructions:

1. Place chicken inside a plastic bag and pound to decrease volume. Wrap 2 slices of bacon around each pounded chicken breasts. They may go around twice. Secure the wrap with a toothpick.

2. When all chicken are wrapped, coat it with olive oil. Rub it around the chicken.
3. In a skillet, use medium heat to cook the chicken. Start with the top side of the chicken facing the pan. Each side of the chicken should take 5-6 minutes to cook.
4. If the chicken is thick, you may stick a thermometer in the thickest part to check if the heat has reached the middle.

### 342. Serve with leafy green salads

This dish tastes great with greens. Use a mix of baby greens like spinach, kale, and chard. Season them with black pepper and sea salt. Use olive oil, cider vinegar, and Dijon mustard with it.

### 343. Serve with paleo coleslaw

Aside from carrot sticks, you can also serve it with simple paleo coleslaw. The tastes from the vegetables should blend well with the meatball.

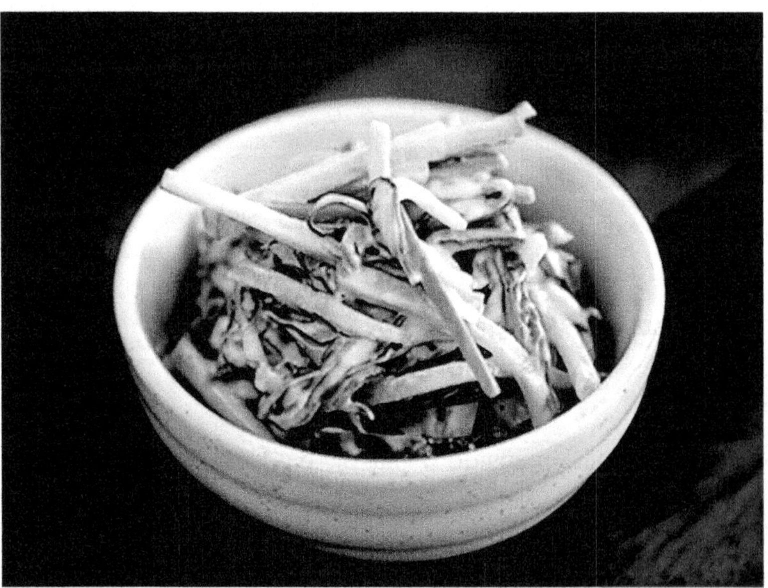

**Photo Source:https://pixabay.com/en/appetizer-background-bowl-cabbage-1223859/**

### 344. Serve with guacamole

You can also use the avocado guacamole suggested in this book with this recipe. You may want to increase the serving of the guacamole to make sure that they are enough for the chicken breast.

### 345. Serve with granola mix cereal

You can also use it as a meat complement to the granola mix cereal recipes suggested in this book. The chicken will add a meaty flavor to those recipes.

### 346. Serve with paleo modified coleslaw

Using paleo-modified coleslaw will also neutralized the salty and fatty flavor of the meats. Use shredded cabbage, carrots, onions, raw honey and apple cider vinegar.

### 347. Serve with fresh ripe fruits

You can also add the cool taste of ripe fruits common in your area. Serve it with a few slices of ripe papayas with coconut milk.

### 348. Rub paprika on the chicken to make it spicier

You can also make a spicy variation of this recipe by rubbing paprika over the chicken before wrapping it with bacon. If you want it to be spicier, let it stand overnight before cooking it.

### 349. Serve with grilled vegetables

This recipe will also go well with grilled bell pepper, tomatoes and Brussel sprouts.

### 350. Serve with sautéed vegetables

If you don’t have time to grill, sauté the vegetables in a pan. You should use ghee or coconut oil for greasing.

### 351. Serve with sautéed onion and mushroom

Aside from vegetables, you can also serve this with caramelized sautéed onions and sliced mushrooms.

### 352. Steamed vegetables with bacon wrapped chicken

Your bacon wrapped chicken meal will be more nutritious if you choose to use steamed broccoli, carrots and green peas.

### 353. Use turkey bacon to cut down on fats

If you are not fond of the fat from the bacon, you can replace it with paleo turkey bacon to wrap the chicken.

# Conclusion

I hope this book was able to help you find paleo recipes that you like. .

The next step is to practice your skills in preparing these recipes and their variations. With continued use of these recipes, you will be able to master ways of mixing ingredients and finding new ways to make healthier and tastier dishes.

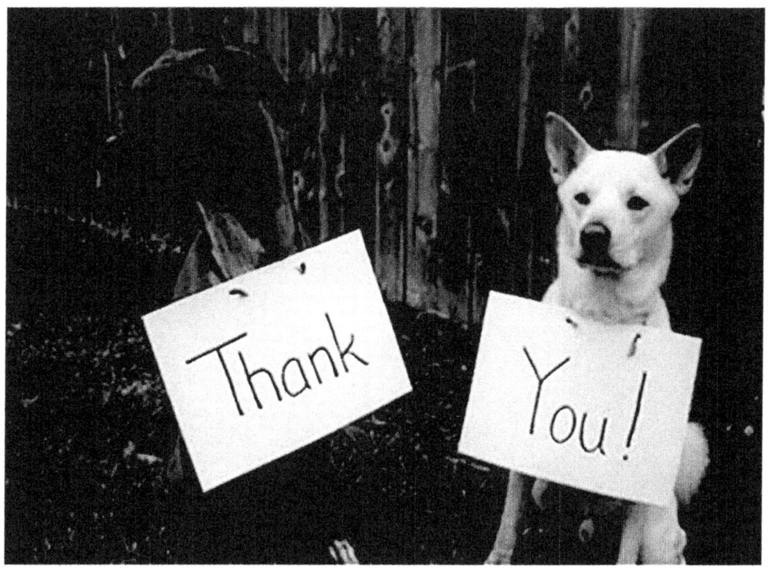


Finally, if you enjoyed this book, then I'd like to ask you for a favor, would you be kind enough to leave a review for this book on Amazon? It'd be greatly appreciated!

Thank you and good luck!

Made in the USA
Middletown, DE
08 April 2022

63866506R00060